Palliative Care in Terminal Illness

SECOND EDITION

James F. Hanratty and Irene Higginson

With a Foreword by

Gill Ford

Radcliffe Medical Press
Oxford and New York

© 1994 Radcliffe Medical Press Ltd
15 Kings Meadow, Ferry Hinksey Road, Oxford, OX2 0DP

141 Fifth Avenue, Suite N, New York, NY 10010, USA

First edition 1989
Second edition 1994

British Library Cataloguing in Publication Data

A catalogue record for this book is available from the British Library

ISBN 1 85775 030 6

Typeset by Tradespools
Printed and bound in Great Britain by
Biddles Ltd, Guildford and King's Lynn

Contents

Foreword

Much has happened in the five years since Dr James Hanratty's *Palliative Care of the Terminally Ill* was first published. This new edition is apposite and welcome – all the more because it comes from such a distinguished and experienced source of medical and nursing care as the St Joseph's team. Much has rightly been said about the contribution that Dame Cicely and St Christopher's have made to the hospice movement, but we must never forget that she spent seven years at St Joseph's, listening to patients and monitoring the development of pain and symptom control. This book, in a sense, is a further progress report from St Joseph's and the nearby Mildmay Unit.

It is part of a widening stream of publications which reflect the much respected art and science of specialist palliative care in the UK, and the growing interest overseas in that development. This volume will be particularly helpful to those making a career in palliative care and seeking a reliable introduction to the field. Those taking initial and in-service courses in a number of professions, apart from nursing and medicine, will also find it most useful; and the same is true for counsellors, clerics and others whose work brings them into the ambit of palliative care.

This is naturally a sphere of work where change is generated both by research and experience, and by the emergence of new problems. This volume reflects that process of change in the excellent contributions by Irene Higginson on symptom control, and in the valuable discussion of AIDS by Veronica Moss. While there is an almost disproportionate research literature on AIDS, if one compares the actual number of cancer and AIDS patients, AIDS is a more recent entrant in the field of palliative care, and one in which the know-how of symptom control is steadily being established and recorded.

The book as a whole, light on the pocket though solid in substance, is to be strongly commended both as a trustworthy introduction and a portable companion for those already established in this field.

Dr. Gill Ford, CB, FRCP
Medical Director
Marie Curie Cancer Care
February 1994

Preface

Most hospices are orientated to the care of patients dying from cancer (which accounts for more than a quarter of deaths in the UK), but the contents of this volume will apply to the care of patients who are dying from whatever cause.

Hospice care is synonymous with palliative care of the highest quality, but it is not the prerogative of hospices; it can be provided equally well in hospitals or in the patient's home. Indeed, the purpose of this book is to be a guide for doctors, nurses and other professional carers in the community just as much as in hospices or hospitals.

The theme of this book may be summarized as 'Compassion with competence'. We all have great compassion for our patients but this needs to be supplemented by practical intervention to provide relief from their distress. Such intervention needs to be given with competence, and this requires some expertise and knowledge of what is available and appropriate, and the capability to apply it efficiently.

The first part of this book is concerned with the philosophy of terminal illness and should assist with the compassionate approach to patient care. The second part is directed towards clinical care and is a guide for the control of distressing symptoms. It is hoped this combination will assist professional carers in their efforts to bring comfort and relief to their patients and to the families.

The first edition of this book was an amalgamation of a series of booklets and papers I had produced to assist teaching doctors, nurses, paramedical carers and students who came to St Joseph's Hospice seeking information on palliative care. Included in this second edition is a chapter on AIDS and HIV by Veronica Moss, the distinguished Medical Director of Mildmay Hospital where patients with AIDS are given superb care.

For assisting me as joint editor, and for largely re-writing 'Control of Distressing Symptoms', I am grateful to Irene Higginson who worked with me at St Joseph's before proceeding to a brilliant career in the wider aspects of palliative care.

To improve the input on nursing care I could do no better than seek the excellent help of the nurses at St Joseph's Hospice, my friends and colleagues for over ten years.

My sincere thanks to my collaborators and also to Gillian Nineham, Editorial Director of Radcliffe Medical Press for her ever helpful guidance; and last but by no means least to my wife, Irene, for her unfailing support and advice.

James F. Hanratty
London, January 1994

I was honoured and delighted when James Hanratty asked me to assist him in preparing this second edition. We have tried to update it to include the many developments in symptom management and psychosocial care for terminally ill patients, including, wherever possible, information which is relevant to cancer and AIDS patients, and those who may have other diseases.

I am extremely grateful to Dr William O'Neill and Dr Beryl McGrath who, at farily short notice, agreed to read and comment on the chapter on the 'Control of Distressing Symptoms'. Their suggestions were extremely valuable in helping me to improve and update this section. My thanks also to Alex Sexton and Franky Eynon for their help in typing the manuscript and to Kate Martin, Editorial Manager, Radcliffe Medical Press, for her helpful guidance.

Irene Higginson

List of Contributors

James F. Hanratty OBE, KSG, MB, ChB, MRCGP
Vice Chairman, Help the Hospices
Formerly Medical Director, St Joseph's Hospice, Hackney, London
- Philosophy of Terminal Illness (except 'The nurse and the dying patient')
(Chapter 1)
- Physiology of Dying (Chapter 4)

Irene Higginson, B Med Sci, BM, BS, MFPHM, PhD
Senior Lecturer and Consultant, Palliative Care Research Group London
School of Hygiene and Tropical Medicine and Kensington, Chelsea and
Westminster Commissioning Agency
- Control of Distressing Symptoms (Chapter 2)

Sister Helena McGilly, RSC, RGN, RM; and Karen Slatcher, RGN, St
Joseph's Hospice, Hackney
- The nurse and the dying patient (Chapter 1)
- Aspects of nursing care included in 'Control of Distressing Symptoms'
(Chapter 2)

Veronica Moss, MBBS DTM&H, DCH, D Obst RCOG
Medical Director, Mildmay Hospital
- Care for Patients with Advanced AIDS and HIV Disease (Chapter 3)

1 | Philosophy of Terminal Illness

'Pray for me, O my friends; a visitant
Is knocking his dire summons at my door,
The like of whom, to scare me and to daunt,
Has never, never come to me before ... '

CARDINAL NEWMAN *The Dream of Gerontius*

Acceptance of the Reality of Death

The prospect of the awesome and inescapable finality of death fills most people with apprehension, fear or even stark terror. The remarkable advances of medicine in the last 50 years have reduced dramatically the numbers of those dying young or in the prime of life; death has largely been deferred to the old and very old and has become relatively remote. This is particularly evident in Western society and has resulted in a death-denying attitude – a sort of naivety whereby death is deliberately not thought of in the hope that by not thinking about it, it will just not happen. Increasing materialism and the diminution of religious interests do not always encourage the contemplation of one's ultimate fate. Life tends to be lived for the enjoyment of the moment; philosophizing about the future being regarded as unrewarding.

Although most patients are aware of the nature of their illness from its history and remorseless progress, not all are prepared to talk about death. This reluctance must be respected by the carers whilst giving the patient every opportunity to discuss the subject. If the patient can be gently led to talk about the reality of death and express fears about it, much of the tension and anxiety will be alleviated.

The Doctor and the Dying Patient

'To cure sometimes, to relieve often, to comfort always.'

Anon. 15th Century

Despite the expertise of modern medicine, some patients are still dying with unrelieved pain and with distressing symptoms inadequately controlled. It is particularly sad that this should be happening when palliative care can provide so many therapies and medications (and these are readily available) to give patients significant and in most cases complete relief from their suffering.

The management of terminal illness is still of variable quality and much seems to depend on the attitude of the professional carer. At one end of the attitude spectrum there are those who would say 'sorry there is nothing to be done' and nothing more is done, largely due to lack of knowledge of what can be done. The family watching the uncontrolled suffering will be haunted by these chilling words in their subsequent bereavement.

Such bleak helplessness with its negative approach to terminal illness was commonplace twenty years ago. Terminal illness was rarely even mentioned in medical training and tended to be regarded as an embarrassing medical failure; doctors by tradition and training being conditioned to do their utmost to achieve a cure. The consequence of this attitude is a distancing between patient and doctor – a cruel deprivation at the one time when a close supporting relationship is crucial. The sense of isolation felt by the patient and their family increases fear, and the constantly changing symptoms of the advancing disease being inadequately controlled means suffering is inevitable.

At the other end of the attitude spectrum there are those doctors who continue to apply vigorous curative treatment, often involving sophisticated 'high-tech' medicine, long after it is obvious that the patient is dying, in a futile bid to keep the patient alive at all costs. Patients and families understandably have a genuine fear of the indignity of this type of treatment. It is never easy to determine exactly when to discontinue efforts to cure, and each patient poses individual problems. The final decision requires consultation with the family, medical and nursing colleagues, and if possible with the patient; indeed not infrequently it is the patient who will decide.

The philosophy of care in terminal illness as developed and promulgated by hospices may be defined: 'the diagnosis having been confirmed, a time comes in the advanced stage of progressive incurable disease such as cancer or AIDS, and death being certain and approaching, when further attempts to cure become irrelevant, unkind, and indeed, bad medicine. A change of role and attitude is then required in the continuing management of the illness by all those caring for the patient.' There is nothing more to be done to *cure* but there is an enormous amount to be done in continuing *care* to ensure that the remaining few weeks or months of the patient's life are spent in comfort and are free from mental and physical suffering.

As a guide in adopting the new role it is helpful to step back and regard the patient as a whole person; but also a person with many facets:

- **Body**: its functions and feelings, its physiology and, especially in terminal illness, the detailed pathological process.
- **Character and personality**: these are remarkably consistent throughout

life. They can however act as a veneer concealing or distorting underlying feelings and fears.

- **Past:** memories, family, education, culture, religion.
- **Present:** 'What's happening to me and my family? Are there things to be done to set my affairs in order?'
- **Future:** 'What is going to happen to me and my family? Will I become dependent, disfigured, a nuisance, be able to cope, lose my mental powers?'
- **Secret life:** we all have fears, desires, hopes, fantasies that we would feel embarrassed to express openly. Psychiatrists and psychoanalysts may probe into these for therapeutic purposes, but it is not appropriate to invade the secret life in the vulnerable state of terminal illness.
- **Transcendant dimension:** even with no formalized religious belief there is a desire in most people to be part of something greater and more lasting than ephemeral earthly life.

Suffering can be related to any of these. It behoves the doctor and caring staff to consider all these aspects of the patient's persona, and with kindness and gentleness bring all medical skills to bear and so provide relief and comfort. If the patient is comfortable so too will the family be that much more at ease.

The Nurse and the Dying Patient

The philosophy of palliative care is for the patient to have the best possible quality of life until death occurs. The nurse must therefore always remember that a dying person is a living and precious person right up to the very end, and the care given should reflect this. The patient is an individual and therefore has the right to individualized care for all needs and should be treated with courtesy and respect at all times, especially with regard to cultural and religious beliefs. Our aim is to free the patient from any distressing symptoms, physical, emotional, spiritual or social, and to maintain life at its full potential.

> 'Rituals express the collective unconscious of the culture, for which they perform a religious, social or therapeutic function.'
>
> Lily Pincus (1974)

As the patient is usually part of a family or circle of friends, the care of both family and friends is an integral part of the nurses' work while the patient is alive and also following death.

First impressions

The first person to greet the patient is usually a nurse. The patient is often very frightened and anxious at this stage, perhaps realizing for the first time that life is coming to an end. First impressions, therefore, are most important. The nurse should have a warm, welcoming approach, using the patient's full name. Non-verbal communication such as the use of eye contact and touch are very reassuring to an anxious patient.

Initial assessment and planning of patient care

During the first meeting with the patient the nurse will make the initial assessment. The patient is often too weak, tired from the journey or confused to answer questions, and information may need to be obtained from the patient or carers later. The nurse can, however, assess many factors from careful observation. For example, if a patient is in pain, the expression will often show this, even if the patient is unable to communicate feelings verbally. Any distressing symptoms, whether physical, emotional or spiritual should be dealt with immediately, in a calm, unhurried manner.

Once the patient's problems have been identified the nurse then plans the care. If any changes to the usual treatment are thought advisable, these must be discussed fully with the patient before implementation.

It is during the initial meeting that the nurse may be able to assess the patient's level of insight. It is important to give the patient ample time to ask questions, and be prepared to give honest straightforward answers.

Implementation and evaluation of care

The nursing team is in a unique position as it provides 24-hour care for the patient. Symptom control and factors such as food/fluid intake and levels of consciousness need to be monitored. Any changes should be reported to other members of the team and appropriate action taken to ensure the patient's symptoms are well controlled at all times. During implementation of care, its effectiveness should be evaluated and treatment adjusted as necessary.

The dying person often experiences feelings of isolation and loneliness. The nurse can greatly alleviate these feelings by being at the bedside with the patient during this difficult time. As the patient gradually becomes weaker the ability to communicate deteriorates. The nurse should be aware that although the patient is unable to respond, sensations of touch and hearing may be intact and the family at the bedside should be informed accordingly.

The nursing care of the family

In today's society, the nuclear family often live at great distances from each other. The use of the word 'family' is therefore intended to encompass all those, whether families, friends, partners or neighbours who are close to the patient.

Admission to a hospice is an emotional experience for all the family. They have often been trying to provide 24-hour care for someone who is very ill, and they may arrive physically and emotionally exhausted.

The first meeting with the family is extremely important. They should be welcomed and not made to feel in the way. They must be given plenty of time to express any fears and anxieties privately with the nurse, who should be sitting down with them prepared to listen and answer any questions. Families often feel very guilty that they have let the patient down by not being able to continue the care at home. They often need affirmation that they have done everything they possibly could to look after the patient. By taking a history from them and including them in the planning of patient care, where appropriate, they realize they still have a significant role to play.

Throughout the patient's stay the family should be kept fully informed with regular updates on the patient's condition. They should feel that the nurse is available to talk with them at any time. This can be achieved very simply by either greeting them when they arrive at the hospice or acknowledging their presence at the bedside.

This is a very stressful time for anyone close to the patient. Families may express this through a variety of reactions, from numbness or disbelief to extreme distress and anger. The anger may be directed at any number of people, including the nurse who should not feel this is directed personally, but is an indication of the extra support needed by the family.

After the death of the patient the nurse who has known the family should spend time with them quietly away from the ward. If good relationships have been built up during the patient's stay, the nurse is now in a better position to understand and give more support, remembering that people from varying backgrounds and cultures will express their emotions differently. Although many people will want to talk about the person they have just lost, this is not always the case. Non-verbal communication such as touch, or sitting in silent empathy can also be helpful.

At this stage it is often difficult for the family to take in any new information, such as how they register the death. It is therefore useful to either write things down or have leaflets available for the family to take away with them.

The role of the nurse within the multidisciplinary team

All members of the multidisciplinary team are available to give support and advice to both the patient and family and to ensure the best possible care. The role of the nurse is often to co-ordinate this care. As the nursing team provide a 24-hour service, patients and their families will often approach them first with any problems they may have. Examples of this are families who are only able to visit in the evening, or patients whose fears and anxieties are keeping them awake at night. In both these cases the nurse will probably be the most accessible member of the team, and needs to be aware of the facilities that are available to the patient from within the care setting and also from external sources.

Good communication links are essential, within both the nursing and multidisciplinary teams. Detailed reports should be given at handover time to the new nursing shift, and the appropriate members of the multidisciplinary team notified of any changes as soon as possible. Communications are enhanced at formal and informal meetings.

As well as nurses and doctors, the team may also have a social worker or psychologist whose training enables them to provide counselling for patients and families. Practical advice on social security benefits or wills is available from the social worker or welfare benefits officer.

The physiotherapist is another member of the team whose skills can help patients retain their full potential within the limits imposed by their illness. Maintaining independence and mobility for as long as possible contributes to the patient's psychological wellbeing. At this difficult time, patients will often receive much comfort from the visits of a hospital chaplain or their own minister of religion to help meet their spiritual needs.

Volunteer helpers as part of the team are often able to provide social contact and distractions, either by enabling the patient to make external visits or by sitting quietly or talking with them. As they are often only present for a few hours a week, the nurse must ensure they are informed of any significant changes and that they are given adequate support.

The individual qualities of the nurse

'What sort of people find themselves called to accompany the dying? At the psychological level one needs three basic attributes: the first is an intensely down to earth practicality ... the second, an over-sized sense of humour ... the third quality is a very special sort of sensitivity: a vulnerability to the pain of others that is often, but not always, the result of personal experience of suffering.'

Sheila Cassidy (1988)

The ability to form supportive relationships not only with patients and families but also with other colleagues is very important. Nurses new to palliative care or younger nurses may never have come into contact with death and dying before. The more experienced nurse should be available to give support and help the new nurse feel more secure. Too often it is seen as a sign of weakness to show emotion and nurses may often bottle up their feelings instead of expressing them to others. There should be opportunities for nurses to discuss difficult and upsetting experiences amongst themselves during informal support sessions, and a staff counsellor should be available for confidential meetings with all members of staff who need extra support.

Maguire and Faulkner[1] talk about the difficulties of looking after dying patients. They suggest these should be acknowledged and dealt with more openly as the emotional price may be too high for the individual.

Nurses must be aware of the importance of relaxation and spending time on other interests when away from work. Senior nurses can be sensitive to these needs by giving reasonable off duty time and trying to meet requests for specific holidays and days off whenever possible. The provision of good orientation programmes and courses in palliative care will improve the nurse's knowledge and confidence. The English National Board (ENB) 931 course in the 'Care of the Dying Patient and their Family', is usually undertaken by those nurses working in this field.

Good communication is essential in all aspects of palliative care. Too often the nurse is made to feel that talking to the patient or sitting quietly with the family is not enough. In palliative care, however, the nurse must learn to develop communication and listening skills as much as a knowledge of symptom control. Stedeford[2] states that communication problems cause more suffering than any other problem except unrelieved pain.

The experienced nurse needs the skills to teach others, whether patients, families or other colleagues, and must keep up-to-date on current issues and be well informed about any new methods of symptom control, attending relevant study days and seminars where possible. The ENB 998 course in 'Teaching and Assessment' can be very helpful to the nurse at this stage.

All nurses providing clinical care need to feel supported by management. By maintaining adequate staffing levels, management can help nurses to provide good palliative care. Praise for a job well done should not be overlooked and can be a tremendous boost for flagging morale. Nursing in palliative care, although rewarding, is very demanding both physically and emotionally. The nurse may find that religious beliefs or life philosophy are a great help and support for this work.

Care of the Dying Patient

'I went to sleep; and now I am refreshed
A strange refreshment; for I feel in me
An inexpressive lightness, and a sense
Of freedom, as I were at length myself ... '

CARDINAL NEWMAN *The Dream of Gerontius*

Effective care of the patient during the last few weeks or months of life requires compassion, competence and constant attention to detail, with every aspect of the patient's condition being studied. The dying patient is still a living person and needs to be treated as such.

Symptoms causing distress need to be discovered, anticipated and then relieved by effective therapy. The threshold at which these symptoms, especially pain, cause distress varies widely. It is personal to each individual and the social, cultural, religious and ethnic background each play a part. It may however fluctuate from day to day – even hour to hour. It is, for instance, lowered if a patient is uncomfortable, tired, worried, afraid, angry or isolated; and conversely it is raised by sympathy, rest, understanding and a pleasing environment.

Patients therefore benefit by being given the opportunity for leisure activities compatible with their condition and interests. The loneliness of the bedridden or chair-bound patient needs to be combated with the help of the relatives and relaxed, unhurried staff. If those around the patient are always busy and in a hurry the patient will be reluctant to complain of discomfort and will refrain from communicating fears and anxieties. Devoted nursing in a bright, colourful environment is essential and the aim should be to give the dependent, vulnerable patient that sense of security which comes from being surrounded with love and kindness.

No two patients are alike and each one needs individual study. It always helps if the purpose of therapy is explained beforehand and the patient's wishes about treatment should be respected. When the patient is first seen, a full medical and social history should be taken and a careful enquiry made about all symptoms (see Appendix 6). A close member of the family should also be interviewed if possible in order to discover any specific problems not mentioned by the patient and also to obtain a fuller knowledge of the patient's personal and domestic background.

An assessment of the patient's insight (knowledge of diagnosis and prognosis) and emotional state should also be made at the first interview.

Symptoms requiring attention in terminal illness are:

Pain	Weakness and tiredness
Dyspnoea	Poor mobility
Cough	Lymphoedema
Nausea and vomiting	Ascites
Intestinal obstruction	Hypercalcaemia
Constipation	Dehydration
Diarrhoea	Haemorrhage
Dysphagia	Excessive sweating
Hiccup	Pruritus
Anorexia	Disfigurement
Cachexia	Smell
Pressure sores	Insomnia
Fungating lesions	Fear and anxiety
Sore and dry mouth	Depression
Urinary problems	Confusion

To control these symptoms the doctor needs to have a comprehensive knowledge of clinical medicine and pharmacology as well as being vigilant for the constantly changing symptomatology accompanying the advancing disease. Symptom control is discussed in detail in Chapter 2 of this book.

As the patient's vital functions begin to disintegrate there is a constant change of symptoms, many of which may be anticipated by a knowledge of the pathological state of the patient. All of these require constant study and application of appropriate medical and nursing procedures to give comfort and to maintain the patient's personal dignity.

It is easy to assume that every symptom causing distress is from the cancer, whereas discomfort may arise from conditions other than the cancer, such as dyspepsia, haemorrhoids, arthritis or toothache, and these should be relieved by appropriate specific treatment.

Patients are all too often given massive doses of tranquillizers or anti-depressant drugs which render them dull, apathetic and drowsy. It is good policy to avoid the use of these drugs unless they are absolutely necessary as the aim is to keep patients alert, lively, active and congenially occupied for as long as possible.

Depression in terminal illness may occur especially in patients who have a history of psychiatric illness. It may also affect patients whose terminal phase lasts many months. These patients may need antidepressants, but depression is not a very frequent feature of terminal illness – about 10 to 15%. Sadness, which is often confused with depression, is an understandable emotion and is not helped by drugs at all. It is best treated by avoidance of isolation, interesting diversion and frequent opportunities for talking with the staff and supportive relatives, and, if appropriate, their pastors.

Whatever therapy is administered to the patient in terminal illness, the doctor should ask him or herself these questions:

- Is this treatment really necessary for the patient at this time, ie is its purpose to give comfort and control distressing symptoms?
- Has the treatment any undesirable side effects or complications? If so, can these be anticipated or minimized?
- Is the treatment of sufficient importance to warrant a full explanation of its implications to the patient and/or relatives, giving them an opportunity to express an opinion with the option to accept or reject the treatment?

Communication in Terminal Illness

It is essential to keep the lines of communication open between the patient, doctor, staff and relatives. This can be done by regular meetings attended by the entire staff, social workers and chaplains, where discussion about patients and families who are posing problems can take place. Sometimes there may be concern about a patient who has particular needs or about relatives who are showing signs of strain and are in need of special support. The relevance of some therapeutic procedures may also need discussion.

Patients frequently present a different face to the various people caring for them and visiting them. They may, for instance, wish to present themselves as a 'good' patient to the doctor and make no complaints when the doctor enquires. But when the doctor has gone, they may be more forthcoming to the nurse or perhaps only to a particular person with whom they have developed some rapport. A complete picture of the patient will only emerge from a combination of the impressions of all those who are caring for them.

These meetings are mutually supportive and all present have the opportunity to express their feelings as regards care of the patients and families. Good team communication enables care to be well co-ordinated, and good communication with patient and family defuses fear, misunderstanding and tension.

When patients and relatives need to have a chat, doctors and nurses should give generously of their time and never be in a hurry or indicate that they have a pressing engagement elsewhere. Time is one of the most valuable things we can give to our patients. Their time is running out and it is so important to enable them to make the most effective use of the time that is left.

Communication with the Patient

'I would have nothing but to speak with thee
for speaking's sake. I wish to hold with thee
Conscious communion; though I fain would know
A maze of things, were it but meet to ask ... '

CARDINAL NEWMAN *The Dream of Gerontius*

Communication with a dying patient is not easy – it is full of emotional hazards and very time consuming. It is not surprising that it is often avoided. Indeed not long ago it was regarded as tantamount to malpractice to divulge to a patient that their illness was terminal. All kinds of subterfuge were adopted to avoid the issue, as it was thought that no patient could accept such devastating knowledge. It was regarded as being both kindly and ethical to use any means, however devious, to avoid telling the patient the truth. Patients were too often fobbed off with facile reassurances.

Times have changed and modern society is much more enquiring and less prepared to take things on trust. However, when it comes to discussion of death there still persists that reluctance to give the patient any opportunity to come to terms with it. Doctors, nurses, families and friends still feel in many instances that they should shield the patient, and they unite in erecting a communication barrier. It is a flimsy barrier because so often they know the patient knows that the illness is terminal, and the patient knows that they know. This situation is perpetuated by constant avoidance of all reference to the patient's prospects. Conversation with the patient is kept on a superficial plane of banality and hollow cheerfulness.

People do not know what to say and are afraid of saying the wrong thing and their kindly sensitivity can lead to reticence. Little do they know that the majority of patients are eagerly awaiting the opportunity to talk about everything that is happening and in prospect. If this is denied them the consequent loneliness adds enormously to their emotional isolation and apprehension.

Given a setting of easy and confident communication, seriously ill people make fewer complaints. If they are given the opportunity, they are only too willing to tell anyone prepared to listen what it is they fear, and if their anxiety can be settled then their pain tolerance can be raised and a reduction of analgesic drugs often follows. Moreover, a spirit of frankness adds a new dimension to the relationship.

There are some patients who prefer not to discuss such matters – although virtually certain of the true prognosis. This reserve and the patient's unexpressed wish must be respected.

There are four guidelines in talking to patients:

1 Listen with care
2 Always be truthful
3 Patients have an absolute right to be told whatever they wish to know about their diagnosis and prognosis, if they ask. They should be given ample opportunities to ask
4 They also have an absolute right *not* to have information thrust upon them which they are not seeking

It needs time, patience and experience to identify the patient's wishes.

At the end of the first interview an open and frank relationship can be initiated by the doctor saying 'Well, I have been asking all the questions so far, have you anything at all you want to ask me?' This gives the patient an early opportunity to achieve a rapport with the doctor and the response may be:

> 'What is the matter with me?'
> 'Will I get better?'
> 'I suppose it must be something serious'
> 'No thanks, I've nothing special to ask'

The last response does not mean that on a later occasion another initiative will receive the same response. It means that the patient at that time is not prepared to risk putting anxieties into words. Further opportunities should be given to the patient from time to time and once rapport is established the patient is much more likely to be responsive.

The doctor should always answer truthfully, but instead of giving the truth harshly or unadorned it is better when answering the questions to turn them around and reply for instance, 'You have asked me that but before I answer, could you tell me what you yourself think about your condition?' It is often helpful at this stage to take the patient through the history of the illness step by step. They are usually well aware of the significance of certain symptoms, for example coughing or vomiting of blood, loss of weight, followed by a battery of tests, operations, radiotherapy and continuing ill-health. In this way most patients are able to work it out for themselves. The doctor should explain in simple, non-technical terms the nature of the illness and the prognosis.

It is impossible to soften the impact of bad news. However it is important to let the patient determine the pace of the discussion. Perception of the implications takes time and the response may be very slow; it should be awaited quietly and patiently.

'How long have I got?' is a frequent question and is difficult to answer accurately. It is very unwise to give a fixed time, eg three months, six months etc. These estimates may occasionally be correct but more often they prove to have been wildly inaccurate, to the embarrassment, and sometimes the distress, of all concerned.

It is kinder therefore to err on the optimistic side when giving a prognosis. Temporary remissions may occur, and even complete regressions, though very rare, are not unknown. A mention of these, emphasizing their rarity, gives that small grain of hope.

Hope indeed is relative to the circumstances. The big hope of course is for a complete cure and restoration to normal good health. Such hope is unrealistic and the patient knows this. There are however many little hopes and these can achieve great importance in the patient's day to day life, for example, hope for a family visit, hope to live long enough for a family celebration such as a birthday or anniversary, or hope for a weekend at home.

What is quite reprehensible is the creation of spurious hope by deliberately misleading the patient. The result of this is often disastrous.

Once the patient has achieved insight into the diagnosis and prognosis there follows a series of supplementary questions to be answered and anxieties to be resolved. The patient may not be able to absorb everything on the first occasion and frequent contacts afterwards are essential. Non-verbal communications assist the development of a harmonious relationship – sitting down beside the patient, showing no indication of being in a hurry and giving full attention to everything discussed. Patients with terminal illness often feel the need for tangible contact with those caring for them, and shaking and holding hands gives physical expression to the personal relationship.

Communication is a two-way process that requires not only give but take. Listening is a special type of skill.

- 'listen with your eyes' – observe gestures, mannerisms, facial expressions
- 'listen with a third ear' – notice any hesitation, omission, intonation
- 'listen attentively' – don't let your mind wander, don't interrupt or provide help if there is hesitation
- don't abhor silence – sitting quietly in silence is immensely supportive.

The rapport achieved by the attentive listener will provide essential information which would be lost by the dreamy passive listener.

A glance back after leaving the bedside is most instructive, as the patient's facial expression at that moment gives an uninhibited indication of the emotional state. A worried, frightened, anxious expression necessitates a return to the bedside as a patient in that state should not be left alone.

Case history

Mrs R. a frail but alert old lady in her early seventies, was admitted with a diagnosis of inoperable carcinoma of the stomach. She had suffered for many years from severe rheumatoid arthritis for which she had been given a series of drugs – some of which have now been withdrawn due to their toxicity. Severe dyspepsia had led her to have a barium meal and the radiologist had reported this as showing a large, craggy ulcer in the lesser curvature typical of a malignant gastric ulcer. As there was a clinical suspicion of liver irregularity, and she was too frail to be subjected to surgery, no further investigations – not even endoscopy were performed. As she lived alone she was referred to the hospice for terminal care. She had already been told that she was suffering from a cancer and had accepted this with resignation.

On admission she was vomiting, nauseated and had intermittent epigastric pain, but no induration was found. She was treated with Ranitidine 150 mg twice daily and she was also given Nystan oral suspension for thrush. With supportive nursing and suitable nutrition her condition began to improve, she gained weight and the dyspepsia cleared. In view of her continual improvement over the following few months she was referred for re-investigations. A repeat barium meal was reported as normal and there was no sign of any malignancy. We had the pleasant task of informing her that she was free from cancer and after arranging for community support she was eventually discharged home.

While we do not wish to subject a patient to a battery of investigations, some of which could be unpleasant, in order to confirm the diagnosis, this case illustrates the pitfalls in accepting a diagnosis from inadequate investigations.

Case history

Mr L. had developed cancer of the nose – a most unpleasant and distressing form of malignancy. In his case it had resisted all attempts at curative treatment and on admission the large fungating tumour had destroyed the central part of his face causing gross distortion and disfigurement and giving the appearance of a gargoyle. A man of sensitivity he was embarrassed and withdrawn and wished to be isolated, but we soon found that behind this revolting 'mask' there was a person of high intellect with a sense of humour and a gentle nature. Once we had got used to his thick speech caused by the cancer, conversation was relaxed and enjoyable and it was easy to forget that he had this disease, when relating to the person behind it. Indeed people were often queuing up to talk to him.

Treatment with antibiotics, including metronidazole for foul-smelling anaerobic infection, Nystan for thrush, morphine and carbamazepine for the pain, made him much more comfortable, and when steroids were added there was a significant reduction of the size of the tumour.

His history was interesting. He and his mother and sister were in a prison camp in Poland during the war. His mother and sister disappeared, but he was spared as he was only twelve years old. Eventually he came to London and became apprenticed as a watch repairer. Later he had a business of his own and married – there were no children. Sadly his wife died and he was left with no known relatives, but he became engrossed in his work and had many intellectual interests. After several months he was happily settled in the hospice with the cancer quiescent. One day he was visited by some 'friends' and following their visit his whole demeanour changed – depressed and withdrawn. Apparently these 'friends' had said 'Oh dear! You must have led a wicked life for God to have punished you in this dreadful way'. Utterly distraught he told them that he had led an average sort of life and never thought of himself as wicked. From being content and indeed cheerful this visit had a destructive effect on his morale and he became despondent and withdrawn. 'There must be something in what they said', was his comment. Although he responded to our efforts he was never able to regain his previous cheerful attitude. He died in his sleep a few months later.

This case history illustrated the damage that thoughtless remarks can cause to patients in terminal illness.

The Reactions and Fears of the Dying Patient

'Now that the hour is come my fear is fled;
And at this balance of my destiny,
Now close upon me, I can forward look
With a serenest joy.'

CARDINAL NEWMAN *The Dream of Gerontius*

Once the patient realizes that death is not too far distant it is essential to give ample time and opportunity for discussing the implications of this realization. Depending on the patient's religion and expressed wishes, the ministrations of a spiritual adviser should be arranged. Even if religious interests have lapsed, a renewal at this time can bring comfort and peace. A legal adviser may also be necessary to provide for an orderly disposition of material assets, and a social worker to help with domestic affairs.

Complete insight does not necessarily imply complete acceptance. Some patients do accept the knowledge of their impending death with quiet resignation and complete placidity. Others however, may have a kaleidoscope of changing emotions and it is important for those caring for the patient to be prepared for these emotions.

Denial

This may follow any temporary improvement. The patient rejects thoughts of dying and erects a mental barrier of denial. There may be talk about the future in unrealistic terms, but it is better not to argue as the denial is the patient's way of coping.

Anger

This may be expressed by constant grumbling and complaining, by spiteful aggressive behaviour and may be directed at anyone – family or staff. Patients showing real anger tend to be regarded as 'awkward people' and may become isolated. Staff and relatives find them difficult to deal with, and not relishing having to accept the patient's anger with tolerance, close and frequent contacts are avoided. The only effective way to help is to grasp the nettle of anger by encouraging an outpouring of emotion, and to kill that anger by demonstrating kindliness and love at all times by all who are in contact with the patient.

Guilt

This is a form of self torture which adds enormously to the sadness of a dying patient. Brooding over past misdeeds, real or imaginary may lead to thoughts that the present situation is a just punishment. Perpetuation of this brooding may lower the symptom threshold and exacerbate the physical suffering. Those caring for the patient should be alert for any evidence of feelings of guilt and not hesitate to seek opportunities to explore them in detail.

Blaming

Seeking a scapegoat may lead to unfair blaming which is often directed towards those who have done most for the patient, such as the family or doctors and nurses. Sometimes previous working conditions or even hospital investigations and surgery are blamed. Patients and their families may become quite obsessed about blaming and may even consider litigation. A full, frank and detailed explanation in simple terms is the most effective way of defusing the situation.

Sadness

This occurs when contemplating the loss of everything one has worked for; loss of family contacts and friends. It is a common and understandable emotion and the patient may appear morose and withdrawn giving the impression that this is really depression. Medication is of no benefit for this; but opportunities to talk and express feelings frankly will give enormous help. Support and frequent contacts with family and friends are of great benefit. *See* case histories pages 75 and 76.

Depression

This is a less common reaction. It is more likely to occur in patients with a history of psychiatric instability and frequently responds to treatment with anti-depressants, but using the smallest effective doses.

The patient's mood ranges through these emotions, oscillating from one to another, and often varying from day to day; with hope intervening. The emotions of the relatives often follow a similar pattern.

Once the reality of impending death is accepted various attitudes towards death may develop.

Death as a friend

This applies particularly to those with faith in a god. They may be able to face death with equanimity, as a homecoming and as a release from the tribulations of this world. There are however those who have no belief in any existence beyond this life and some of these may be capable of achieving an inner peace too. Others who regard death as a friend are those who feel that they have obtained what they could out of their lives and are now able to face death with fatalistic acceptance.

Death as an enemy

This affects those for whom the prospect of forced separation from all that is familiar, and from loving and intimate relationships leads to a feeling of utter desolation and loneliness. They become angry, bewildered and terrified and need constant support from the whole caring team.

Death as a challenge

This is similar to when the alarm is sounded for action stations in wartime. There is the prospect that something unknown is going to happen very soon and the ultimate outcome is uncertain. The feeling of apprehension is compounded with a determination to do one's duty with dignity – not to let oneself or others down, and to accept with resignation whatever may be the outcome.

Death the indignity

The fear of many is the prospect of pain unrelieved, the embarrassment of incontinence, the frustration of immobility and the dread of irrationality. The patient should be given ample time to express these fears, and needs to have confident reassurance of constant caring support.

Most people however do not formulate their feelings so rigidly. Equanimity may be sought by discussing these fears with a member of the caring team, with a relative, sympathetic friend or with a spiritual adviser. A patient should be encouraged to look for some goal of pleasure and enjoyment in each day:

> A visit from a friend today
> I went out into the garden today
> My favourite football team won today

Sometimes it helps to keep a diary recording each day's pleasures. Many patients sitting quietly and thinking need some guidance and it helps to give them themes for meditation:

> What have I done with my life?
> What achievement(s) can I look back on with satisfaction?
> Is there anything I really wish to do now before I become weaker?
> Whom do I really love and cherish?
> Who really loves and cherishes me?
> What does death mean to me?

For those who have a religious faith – prayer and contemplation, and arranging meetings with their religious pastors can assist in achieving spiritual peace and tranquillity.

A patient should be encouraged to be as busy as possible with enjoyable activities: reflecting on happy memories – holidays, family celebrations or achievements; browsing through a family photograph album; meditating on religious or spiritual themes. The consolation and comfort patients obtain will depend largely on the religious, cultural, social and ethnic influences in their lives.

Providing patients with opportunities for diversion and creative activities gives them great pleasure and a sense of fulfilment. There is no doubt that it also raises their symptom threshold. Physical condition and personal interests will determine what is appropriate, although many patients gain great skill and enjoyment by taking up activities of which they had no previous experience. *See* case histories pages 32 and 75. Some prefer to participate in group activities and others would rather be alone and concentrate on individual interests. Computer chess can be quite absorbing.

Efforts undertaken in providing diversion are supremely worthwhile and there are all kinds of gadgets designed to assist those with special disabilities (*see* Disabled Living Foundation Appendix 1). Especially rewarding are visits to shops, cinema, theatre, the local pub and country drives. These all help patients to feel that they are still part of the pattern of daily life.

The arts, too, are important, books, music, writing, painting, needlework. (For help with 'talking' books, tapes, music – *see* Appendix 1.) As there is much time for quiet reflection some patients find comfort in expressing their feelings in poetic terms when they would find it too difficult to put these feelings into words.

Pets are often an integral part of a family and some people are greatly saddened by the separation from their pet when admitted to in-patient care. This should be recognized and contacts encouraged. A well behaved hospice dog or cat becomes a great favourite.

An evening round of drinks will provide a relaxed social atmosphere, but patients should not be pressurized into attending.

The objective is to enable patients to *live* until they die and not merely to exist.

Communication with the Relatives

> 'What is termed the "agony of death"
> concerns the watcher by the bedside
> rather than the one who is the subject of pity.'
>
> SIR FREDERICK TREVES

From the time the patient is admitted the close co-operation of the family should be sought as an essential contribution to the totality of care. The contact should continue throughout the illness to the death of the patient and extend through the bereavement for as long as it is needed. This may be for months or occasionally years.

The interview with the relatives at the time of admission, when salient information concerning the patient is obtained, also gives an opportunity to develop a friendly association. Frequent contact afterwards should be encouraged and can be facilitated by having flexible visiting times. The patient's illness often incurs family, financial or domestic difficulties, and the help of a knowledgeable and sympathetic social worker may bring considerable comfort to the often confused and frightened family.

Sometimes the family have a sense of guilt because the patient can no longer be kept at home. Often there have been prolonged and heroic efforts to continue the home care, and the relatives are greatly relieved to be reassured that the time has now come when in-patient care is essential.

Many relatives obtain much needed comfort by being allowed and encouraged, under guidance, to perform or assist with some parts of the nursing care. They can give practical and often very useful assistance, which is much appreciated by the patient and staff.

Case history

Mr A. aged 29 had a cerebral tumour. Weak and drowsy he needed total nursing care. Angela his young wife, a schoolteacher, came straight from school remaining with him during all her spare time, holding his hands and weeping inconsolably. At a ward meeting it was decided to involve Angela in her husband's care by leaving the simpler nursing procedures for her to do. The transformation was dramatic. She came bustling into the ward busily taking over from the nurses and her whole demeanour was changed so that soon she was helping with the care of other patients too. After her husband's death she was a frequent visitor. Knowing that she had been able to take an active role in her husband's care was a great comfort in her bereavement.

It is sometimes helpful to give relatives a few guidelines on visiting. Too many people should not visit at the same time, and there is no need for constant talk – especially the sort of talking which requires a response from the patient.

Sitting quietly, holding the patient's hand and enjoying the contact in silence, may seem strange at first but, once achieved, visits made in this way give great mutual comfort.

The understandable protectiveness of the relatives may extend to their desire to shield the patient from all knowledge of the diagnosis and prognosis. 'You won't tell will you doctor?' It is necessary at an early stage to point out that it is the patient who should decide, and that the doctors and nurses are not prepared to enter into a conspiracy of deceit (*see* Communication with the patient, page 10). At the same time, the relatives should be reassured that any discussion with the patient will be conducted in a gentle, soothing and supportive manner, and they will be kept fully informed.

Frequently the doctor and nurse are able to act as catalysts between the patient and relative to achieve an openness and ability to discuss the implications of the terminal illness. The consequent release of tension is a great comfort to everyone.

> 'It is incredible how much happiness
> even how much gaiety, we sometimes
> had together after all hope of recovery
> was gone. How long, how tranquilly,
> how nourishingly, we talked together
> that last night!'
>
> C. S. LEWIS *A Grief Observed*

Bereavement

> 'No one ever told me that grief felt so like fear.
> I am not afraid, but the sensation is like being afraid.
> The same fluttering in the stomach, the same restlessness ... '
>
> C. S. LEWIS *A Grief Observed*

The death of a loved one inflicts grievous pain on those who were near and dear, and the pain is none the less, even if the death came as no surprise. The initial reaction is a feeling of numbness, disbelief, and even a denial that this can really have happened.

After the first few days of shock there develops an awareness of the reality of the death, and subsequent grief may take differing and fluctuating forms in various combinations.

Anger

This is very frequent with a desire to throw things about and an impatience and irritability with everyone, even with those who are doing their best to help.

Guilt and blaming

This involves a recapitulation of the events leading up to the death, and an analysis of these events. 'If only I had done so and so this would not have happened.' Self-castigation leads to the agony of remorse. These thoughts can easily lead to blaming others, 'If only *they* had done so and so, this would not have happened.' The sad thing about this train of thought is that very often those who have done the most to help, such as members of the family, doctors and nurses, are deeply hurt by this 'blaming'.

Disorganization

This often follows due to lack of interest and unwillingness to apply the mind to the mundane requirements of day to day life.

Isolation

A withdrawal from social contacts may be due to a feeling of embarrassment at causing others to feel uncomfortable should an attack of uncontrollable weeping occur. There is also the awkwardness of conversation even with close friends; an artificiality and superficiality when people constantly try to avoid any reference to the one subject that is uppermost in everyone's mind. The sensation of being an object of pity when appearing in public makes many people prefer to isolate themselves from friends and neighbours. Another cause of isolation is that they just cannot be bothered to make the effort to go out and about.

There is a significant increase in the morbidity and mortality of widows and widowers during the first year of bereavement as compared with those of similar age and background who have not been bereaved. This may well be due to self-neglect and isolation, or a diminished will to overcome adversity.

The Care of the Bereaved

'Blessed are they that mourn: for they shall be comforted.'

Matthew 5:4

The general demeanour of those visiting the dying patient during the last few weeks should be observed discreetly by the caring staff. This will give some indication of those who are likely to need some further support during bereavement. The social worker and those involved in bereavement care should be alerted and briefed and follow-up visits made. These visits may have to continue over months or even years depending on the amount of support which is found to be necessary.

Anticipatory care may often diminish the intensity of subsequent grief, by giving every possible support to those visiting the dying patient; by ensuring that the patient's distressing symptoms are effectively controlled; and by having an affectionate relationship with the patient and the family. The bereaved will then be able to look back and re-live those stressful weeks with some satisfaction.

'After all the death was so peaceful'
'Everything possible was done'

The funeral is not the grand finale. The next day is normal for others, but not for the bereaved and it is difficult to adjust to life as a half of a Mr and Mrs, or without a partner, parent, child or other close relative or friend. They have lost a companion, a sexual partner, a mother/father of children and a confidante.

The most effective way to help the bereaved is to achieve a relaxed relationship whereby it becomes easy to talk freely about the one who has died. Let the bereaved person talk, and talk uninhibitedly about anything and everything connected with the one who has died. Dwelling on family memories, looking at old photographs, and having someone available to listen sympathetically are some of the ways of obtaining comfort and consolation. It is important to avoid platitudes such as: 'Time will cure', 'Go away for a holiday to help you forget', 'Don't keep dwelling on it all'. These are meaningless and can be hurtful.

Grief is the price paid for love and if it could all be forgotten so easily by the passage of time, by having a holiday, by not dwelling on it, that loving relationship must indeed have been fragile and without substance. The passage of time helps to assuage the grief but will never eradicate it; the scar will always remain.

The purpose then, in caring for the bereaved, should be to achieve reintegration rather than substitution.

The use of drugs such as tranquillizers and antidepressants conspicuously fails to give more than ephemeral comfort to the bereaved. Occasionally a pathological depression may occur which necessitates psychiatric treatment and the use of antidepressant drugs. Apart from these cases drugs should be prescribed very sparingly in the treatment of the bereaved – perhaps the occasional night sedative in the first few weeks and nothing further. Many people become drug dependent after drugs have been prescribed to treat bereavement.

Much help may be given to the bereaved by putting them in touch with others in a similar situation. CRUSE, the Compassionate Friends and the Samaritans can provide useful support (*see* Appendix 1). Financial advice may also be necessary and the social worker should be able to advise on benefits and welfare rights. Further help can also be obtained from organizations such as Age Concern, One Parent Families and Child Poverty Action Group (*see* Appendix 1).

When appropriate the bereaved should be encouraged to have recourse to their religious faith and seek the guidance of their pastor and the companionship of fellow members of that faith. It may be months, even years, before the bereaved person succeeds in becoming effectively adjusted to everyday life without the support of the one who has died.

> To everything there is a season,
> and a time to every purpose under the heaven:
> A time to be born, and a time to die . . .
> A time to mourn . . .
> A time for peace . . .
>
> Ecclesiastes 3:1–8

Financial problems may add to the burden for many bereaved people, especially if the partner has been chronically sick for some time and has not been able to work. Often people are reluctant to disclose these problems, and gentle probing may be necessary to find out whether the family has sufficient income to pay for the funeral costs, and to live on afterwards.

The hospice social worker, local social services department or the social security office should be able to advise on welfare benefits available. Welfare rights offices or Citizens Advice Bureaux are also able to help when there are legal or financial difficulties.

One very useful leaflet, issued by the Department of Social Security is D49 – *What to do after a death*. This includes practical information on arranging a funeral, what to do with property and possessions and where to get help.

Supplies can be obtained from the local social security office or from the address in Appendix 1.

Home Care

> 'Be it ever so humble, there's no place like home.'
>
> J. H. PAYNE (1792)

Most people if asked where they would prefer to be for their final illness would opt for their own home, provided that essential care would be available. Understandably, patients are more relaxed and more content when they are in the familiar surroundings of their own home and in the presence of their own loving family. About 40 or 50 years ago most patients (about two thirds) did remain at home for their final illness. Now it is the converse and over two thirds of deaths occur away from home – in hospitals, hospices or residential nursing homes.

When it is apparent that a patient is nearing the terminal stage of progressive, incurable illness, a meeting of all interested parties should be held – patient, family, doctor and nurse – to discuss future management and plans. Certain questions require answers.

- What are the patient's wishes?
- What are the carer's/carers' wishes?
- Is the home suitable?
- Are there the necessary amenities, eg heating, bath, lavatory, and are these conveniently accessible?
- Should the patient be moved to another room?
- Who is available to provide the care at home and are they willing, available and capable (if there are several available, make out a rota)?
- Are there good communications such as a telephone? Otherwise what are the plans for obtaining assistance?
- Secure help of community services (*see* Caring for the carers below).
- Are the general practitioner and nursing services able to carry the burden of frequent and sometimes lengthy visits?
- What other support, eg Macmillan nurses or home care support services are available?
- Make advance plans on what to do should home care support break down, or patient and/or carers change their minds and prefer in-patient care.
- Is there an adjacent hospice? In any case contact the nearest hospice to obtain advice on specific problems.
- Consider if it is possible for the patient to attend a hospice for day care and for occasional admissions for special care.
- The local pharmacist should be alerted eg to have appropriate stock levels of opioids, and for assistance in compliance by clear explanation when supplying the drugs.

At the initial meeting a detailed protocol of liaison should be agreed between a palliative home care team and the GP and community nurses team. It is especially important to decide who is to do the prescribing in order to avoid confusion caused by multiple prescribing from different people. Every hospice has experience of patients being admitted with carrier bags full of large numbers of drugs, all mixed up, and neither patient nor family having the faintest idea of what they are for and when to take them.

The carers and patient should understand clearly what medication is being given and what it is for. A chart listing all medication with times of dosage should be left in the house. Medical and/or nursing notes left in the house should be simple and clear so that someone unfamiliar with the patient will be able to provide appropriate treatment. Carers must always be kept fully informed about treatment, and ample time should be given to answer their queries and give them the support they need.

While transfer to in-patient care may become necessary and the correct decision, it is always a traumatic experience if this is deferred until the last moment when the patient is '*in extremis*' and may die on the journey, or shortly after in-patient transfer. 'Last minute' panic admission to in-patient care may be pre-empted by earlier discussions with the resident carers. They will be given confidence by firm assurance that doctors and/or nurses are always available for visiting. Marie Curie nurses giving domiciliary care are a great comfort – especially during the night. Perhaps the most important aspect of home care is continuity of care by the same team of doctors and nurses. Emergency visits from total strangers are a poor substitute.

Always visit when the patient dies. The patient is beyond our care but the bereavement support for the family is just beginning. It is important to remember that in home care the roles are reversed from in-patient care. Doctor and nurse are the visitors; patient and family the hosts. Appropriate courtesies should always be observed.

Caring for the Carers

This is a rough translation of the Latin phrase, 'Quis custodiet ipsos custodes', which indicates that it is an age-old problem; indeed it is a problem as old as human life itself. Sadly, its importance is still frequently unrecognized.

The carer at home

Since the last war there have been fundamental changes in our Western society resulting in smaller families, dispersed families, more women working outside the home and different social attitudes. An illness at home can have serious consequences for the carer who may try to continue with an outside job for fear of losing it. Many homes are run on a financial 'knife-edge' and loss of income is disastrous.

The carer at home is usually a woman – mother, daughter, or an in-law, and occasionally no relation at all, eg a kindly landlady or neighbour. The professional carers such as doctors, nurses, social workers, however devoted, are just short-term visitors to the home, and the continuing strain of coping with a seriously ill person inevitably rests with the resident carer, often with no respite.

The effect of the unrelenting responsibility will soon lead to various forms of tension. The carer will feel isolated, unable to enjoy normal social activities and have a diminished quality of life. Loss of sleep and ordinary relaxation will affect general health and eventually lead to reduced sympathy towards the patient and consequent feelings of guilt. The professional carers must be aware of these incipient problems and anticipate them by providing appropriate support from the beginning such as:

- teaching the simpler nursing procedures
- improve carer's morale by praising good care
- reassurance that someone will always be available should anxieties arise, for example where is the nearest telephone if there is none in the home?
- volunteer night support from the local community, eg church, neighbours, etc
- arranging a night sitter, Marie Curie nurse, Meals on Wheels, laundry service
- periodic attendance at a Day Centre if there is one available and if the patient's condition permits
- respite admissions to local hospice or hospital
- ensuring that all statutory supplementary payments are being received
- trying to arrange that professional care is given by the same people. It is upsetting if total strangers arrive knowing nothing about the circumstances.

The contribution of the social worker is of special importance in home care. Apart from providing comforting personal support, the social worker has knowledge of what is available from the community, statutory and voluntary services and also has the professional ability to deploy these effectively.

The carer in hospice or hospital

If patient care is provided by a team consisting of doctors, nurses, paramedical and social workers, the team should have regular meetings to discuss the care of patients and their families. Patients frequently show a different face to different members of the team, being quiet and reserved to some and chatting freely and uninhibitedly to others. At these meetings all present should be free to express their views about all aspects of patient and family care, and also their own personal attitudes. The meetings also provide mutual support and an opportunity to share with colleagues the stressful aspects of the work.

Other guidelines for staff support

There should be easy and informal access to senior members of the team, eg ward sisters and doctors who should be prepared to give ample time for discussion of problems and tensions.

Effective training should be provided so that staff are fully aware of the philosophy of palliative care. Recreation and leisure activities should be encouraged.

Careful selection of staff is essential. This work is not suitable for those who have had a recent bereavement or a history of emotional instability.

A particular form of stress may manifest itself in those who are closely involved in the care of terminal illness. Variously called 'burn-out' or 'battle fatigue' it arises from problems of communication with patients, families or colleagues resulting in a feeling of isolation and lack of support. Difficulty in coping with special problems in patient or family care, or administrative mismanagement, will add to the stress and lead to self-criticism and a feeling of being inadequate. Those affected are tense, irritable, humourless, and become obsessive about their work. They refuse to take time off and feel that the system will break down without their presence. It is important for the team to be alert for early signs of stress in colleagues. Firm action is needed to restore confidence and self-esteem to those affected and this may well involve transfer to other work.

Ethical Issues in Terminal Illness

Communication

This is dealt with at length in previous chapters. It cannot however be over-emphasized that open and honest communication on all sides is paramount in achieving trust in terminal care. The relationship between doctors, nurses, patient and family is based on trust, it is fostered by friendliness and it is destroyed by deceit or suspicion; and once destroyed it can never be regained.

Prognosis is an inexact art and the short answer should always be 'I don't know', although it will be necessary to qualify this and discuss the patient's condition in more detail. Assessments in terms of days, weeks or months should be avoided. What is quite reprehensible is to tailor the prognosis in over-optimistic terms to suit and please the patient, while giving a completely different prognosis to others.

Refusal of treatment

It is a patient's right to accept or refuse treatment. It is however essential that the patient should realize the implications so that an informed decision can be made. A full and detailed explanation should be given with ample time for discussion. If necessary, further professional opinion should be made available.

Some patients understandably reject chemotherapy or surgery for fear of unpleasant complications. The pros and cons should be set out clearly. A refusal is easier to accept if it is treatment unlikely to produce a cure, or will just provide temporary amelioration at the expense of much discomfort. Patients, because of their illness are essentially vulnerable and should not be pressurized to make a decision which conflicts with their inclinations. However, what is harder for the carers to accept is when a patient refuses treatment which will certainly give comfort and relieve distress, for example, a patient who refuses to have morphine for severe pain. Nevertheless, such a refusal must be accepted if that is the patient's firm and informed decision. The acceptance by the carers of such a decision must be complete and the patient must not be treated with discourtesy for going against the carer's advice. The care staff should not become sulky. Refusal of treatment may be by a patient who is mentally confused or paranoid. Here persuasion may be used and often succeeds. It is quite wrong to disguise drugs and give them surreptitiously, for example in food and drink. If however a patient has a florid psychosis where sedation is vital, it is then justifiable to administer a drug against the patient's wishes as this is for the patient's own safety.

Complementary therapies

It is understandable when patients are suffering from a progressive incurable illness which has not responded to orthodox medicine, that they should seek treatment from unorthodox sources. Such treatment may be anathema or even offensive to the patient's doctor, but provided it is given in good faith and is not likely to do any harm it must be accepted. Indeed, patients would become resentful and unco-operative if they were deprived of treatment which they were convinced might be of some help.

During recent years there has been a proliferation of complementary therapies, many of which are extensions of treatment routinely given in physiotherapy or occupational therapy. Touch techniques, various forms of massage and exercises, aromatherapy, reflexology may provide comforting relaxation. Massage, especially if accompanied by exercises should be given with caution bearing in mind the risk of pathological fractures.

There have been claims of benefit from certain diets and from large doses of vitamins. In general, these are harmless but medical guidance is essential to avoid undesirable side-effects.

Although acupuncture has been used in China since 2000 BC there is still uncertainty about how it works. Recent experiments support the theory that analgesia from acupuncture is mediated by the release of endogenous opioids. Its use for relieving chronic pain merits serious consideration but further investigation is needed. Meanwhile acupuncture in palliative care should be in the hands of doctors (usually anaesthetists) experienced in its use.

Homoeopathy is available within the NHS and while some doctors are convinced of its value in symptom control, many others are puzzled about how it can work. Its theory is to treat 'like with like' ie treating symptoms with drugs which cause similar symptoms but using extremely attenuated doses.

Hypnosis has its adherents and in the hands of an experienced psychiatrist may assist with relaxation and some degree of symptom control.

Exaggerated and unrealistic claims are frequently made regarding the benefits from various types of complementary therapy. As in every aspect of treating dying patients and their families, open communication and discussion are essential, and if complementary therapy is arranged it should be by agreement with the caring team of professionals.

Families have been impoverished by becoming involved in very expensive and often bizarre treatments and it is our duty to protect them from being exploited. Terminal illness makes them extremely vulnerable.

Ordinary and extraordinary treatment

It is the fundamental duty of those caring for the patient to provide at all times what is termed ordinary treatment, and it is the patient's right to have and to expect to be given such treatment. Ordinary treatment is that which is necessary to give comfort to the patient, for example the relief of distressing symptoms by appropriate medication and therapy; kindly, sympathetic nursing care and assistance with natural functions and mobility; provision of, and assistance in taking, adequate nutrition and fluids.

Extraordinary treatment is an aggressive application of therapies over and above ordinary treatment and given in order to achieve a cure or prolongation of life; but at the same time is a treatment which has inherent risks and complications. These need to be balanced against the chances of a successful or acceptable outcome.

Problems of decision arise because what is at one time ordinary treatment may at another time, and in the same patient, become extraordinary treatment. For example, the provision of adequate nutrition and fluids would become extraordinary treatment for the patient in semi-coma whose life is drawing to a close.

Whenever extraordinary treatment is contemplated, it should be preceded by full and frank discussions with everyone concerned – the patient, if this is possible, close relatives, and senior medical and nursing colleagues. There should be full documentation of all discussions and also of the treatment.

Examples of extraordinary treatment include: surgical by-pass for intestinal obstruction due to abdominal carcinomatosis; aggressive chemotherapy and life support resuscitation. This is an issue for which it is impossible to make hard and fast rules as each patient is unique and poses individual problems.

Ethical Problems in Different Ethnic Groups

Communication

Language difficulties pose many problems especially if the patient and family come from ethnic groups with its own language. Every hospice needs to have pictures which can be used in obtaining information from the patient and the family while awaiting the services of an interpreter. It is essential to have a panel of interpreters from whom assistance may be obtained very rapidly. If an uncommon language is met, an approach to the appropriate Embassy will often be successful in obtaining someone knowledgeable in the language. The requirements of the care of patients in terminal illness involve close rapport with patient and family and if this has to be done through an interpreter it can be very time consuming and exhausting for everyone. Nevertheless it is absolutely essential that effective interpretation be achieved so that the patient and the family are fully cognizant of the patient's illness, prognosis and treatment being given, and also able to answer questions and express anxieties and fears.

Occasionally the communication is complicated by an element of distrust which is based on fear, unfamiliarity, and lack of knowledge of the procedures of medical and nursing care in the UK. This can require prolonged and careful discussion in order to eradicate the distrust, and again can be extremely difficult if it has to be done through an interpreter; nevertheless it must be done.

Cultural attitudes may cause problems. For example, there are some ethnic groups where women are not allowed to express any opinions for themselves and the men regard it as their duty to monitor every aspect of care including medical and nursing procedures. This attitude sometimes arouses antagonism in the female staff who resent the fact that the women have been kept so subservient.

Non-acceptance of orthodox medical care

Frequently ethnic groups have been cared for by their own medical and nursing friends, some of whom may have no medical or nursing qualification in this country. There may also be problems of diet which at times complicate and indeed militate against orthodox medical care. Explanation is essential; giving full details of what is involved.

Non-acceptance of the philosophy of hospice care

The philosophy of hospice care as practised in the UK is that the time comes in terminal illness when continued efforts to cure the patient are irrelevant and inappropriate as the patient's condition has extended beyond the stage where cure is possible. Continuing care therefore is concerned with relieving suffering and controlling distressing symptoms as well as emotional support for the patient and the family.

There are some ethnic groups who will not accept this philosophy and insist that the patients are given the equivalent of intensive care right through to the very end. Hospices are not equipped to provide this type of care, and problems, particularly in relation to the family, may result. It is therefore most important to explain to the family the philosophy of hospice care at the very beginning in order to avoid misunderstandings.

Religious and cultural attitudes

The staff of the hospice must at all times be prepared to welcome, inform and as far as possible, co-operate with the legitimate pastors of the patient and family. Sometimes aggressive friends or neighbours may present themselves as representatives of the patients' and families' interests. It is therefore important that pastors should be known as legitimate religious leaders.

The hospice must make itself aware of the religious and cultural attitudes of various ethnic groups with regard to the practices adopted when the patient dies and also with the procedures for the care of the body and its disposal[3]. The hospice should have readily available as much information as possible on these cultural and religious practices.

Disruption may occasionally be caused by these cultural and religious procedures, especially for other patients and their families, eg ritual wailing. In this case a suitable room should be available for patient and family.

Euthanasia

The humanitarian and emotional reaction aroused in those observing someone severely disabled, diseased or dying are understandably distressing – particularly for the family. Not knowing what to do or what to say to alleviate apparent suffering leads to frustration and helplessness. The suffering, in many cases, is on the part of the beholder not the patient.

It is a dreadful indictment of our medical services that one of the main arguments in favour of euthanasia is that some people do die in physical and mental distress. However the patient should not have to be killed in order to stop distress. Patients in terminal illness occasionally, with the agreement of their family, may ask either explicitly or by veiled hints, for an early end to their illness, ie they want the doctor to kill them.

This request should be regarded as a cry for help and it should not be brushed aside or ignored. It is easy to say 'That cannot be done, it is illegal' (which of course it is) and leave it at that. What is essential is to have long and detailed discussions with the patient to identify the problem (or problems) which prompted the request. The usual reason is fear or even terror of the process of dying which is anticipated as being accompanied by unrelieved physical distress such as pain or suffocation. These fears should be explored in depth and can be rapidly dissipated by establishing close rapport, gaining the patient's confidence, giving firm reassurance that symptoms will be relieved, and that someone known and trusted will always be available. Other reasons are loss of self-esteem, a feeling that life is now useless and that they are a burden to everyone, and emotional and spiritual desolation. It is always important to impress on patients that, despite the fact that their condition is such that they are constantly receiving, they are nevertheless unwittingly giving; giving of themselves and of their personalities. We the carers and their family are grateful to them for their presence and for the opportunity just to be with them.

Contact with the religious pastor, encouragement with recreational activities and enhancing personal appearance all help to bring comfort and tranquillity, and counteract the despair underlying the request for euthanasia. The confident reply to such requests is palliative care of the highest quality to enable patients to *live* until they die.

Nevertheless, there are those who with kindly intentions continue to campaign for voluntary euthanasia to be legalized. They do not realize that what they are seeking is veterinary medicine in preference to Hippocratic medicine. Moreover, the unique and inviolable quality of human life is a fundamental tenet of the Judaeo-Christian religion. If euthanasia were to be legalized, some patients out of altruism might suggest it themselves: 'I don't want to be a nuisance'; 'I'm just spoiling their lives'. On the other hand, knowing that euthanasia was permissible patients might begin to suspect their doctor's actions.

Inevitably the attitudes of doctors and nurses would harden, with a diminishing respect for the unique quality of human life. Indeed they might soon start to encourage patients to accept euthanasia (particularly those patients posing difficult medical and nursing problems). Doctors would find themselves conniving at assisted suicide; a socially dangerous and negative approach which confirms the patient's despair and denies all hope.

Euthanasia would be damaging and divisive to the family. Subsequent guilt reactions, accusations, recriminations and dissensions would have serious repercussions throughout the family.

Selecting patients for euthanasia would depend on the accuracy of diagnosis and prognosis. There can be very few doctors and nurses who cannot recall gross diagnostic errors, and many will have had the embarrassing experience of committing themselves to a prognosis which proved to have been wildly inaccurate. (*See* case history, page 13.)

A society accepting euthanasia would soon become a sick society itself. Once it was realized that when a human life became difficult to sustain and could be eliminated by euthanasia, this practice would be encouraged and in the long-term even become mandatory.

After a year of deliberations a British Medical Association Working Party on Euthanasia reported in 1988. Its conclusion was that 'The Law should not be changed and the deliberate taking of a patient's life should remain a crime'.

In a booklet issued by the World Health Organization in 1990, the Expert Committee stated 'With the development of modern methods of palliative care, legislation of voluntary euthanasia is unnecessary'.

Finally, in an address to MPs and Peers in the House of Commons in December 1991, Dame Cicely Saunders concluded 'We need to emphasize to our colleagues and the public that there is an acceptable form of appropriate treatment being researched and taught that needs no laws for its establishment, and that any law such as has been suggested would be dangerous and demeaning to many vulnerable people and finally, impossible to draft without frightening possibilities for abuse'.

Case history

In 1968, Mr E., then aged 38, had a nocturnal fit, was taken to hospital, and after a stormy illness (encephalitis with bulbar palsy) ended with almost complete quadriplegia, dysphagia and aphasia. He had been a pilot officer in the RAF and on demobilization became a sales manager with an electronics firm and was married with two children.

During the early stages, laborious communication was established with the help of his wife and an alphabet board – nodding his head when the correct letter was indicated. On admission to a hospice in 1974 his quadriplegia was complete, apart from weak movements of his right index finger. He could nod his head and was still unable to speak, but his dysphagia was less troublesome. He had experienced periods of profound depression and frustration.

Gadgets were made to maximize his finger movement enabling him to touch type and thereby to communicate. Later he was able to paint with assistance using a palette. He is still in the hospice and his disability is just as profound as when he was admitted, needing comprehensive nursing care and physiotherapy for his quadriplegia and medical care for occasional chest and urinary tract infections.

He has a very busy life, corresponding with numerous friends, has written a book 'The Long Road Back', goes home for most weekends, and with the help of family and friends has had holidays in Portugal and Switzerland. He has painted many very attractive pictures and is experimenting with glass engraving.

In the early days he was devastated at the prospect of life with such a major disability, but having got through that period with the help of his devoted wife and family, he is now enjoying a full, interesting and busy life. He is certainly glad that euthanasia was not available as he would have accepted it eagerly in the early days of his illness.

Advance Directives

Doctors and hospitals, especially in the USA, are increasingly concerned about allegations of malpractice which if successful, often result in awards of enormous damages by the Courts. Doctors caring for patients in terminal illness are especially vulnerable. They are in an invidious position whereby, unless they provide the equivalent of intensive care they may be accused of not trying hard enough, yet, if they do just that they may be blamed for inflicting suffering by prolonging the patient's life unnecessarily. To pre-empt this dilemma many doctors now practise defensive medicine and one device is the Advance Directive.

This is a mechanism whereby a competent person gives instructions about what should or should not be done if the capacity for self-expression should be lost. This enables the patient's autonomy to be preserved by pre-selecting or refusing treatments which might in certain circumstances be proposed and which the patient would not at that time be in a condition to discuss.

While it is always useful to know what patients' wishes are there might be serious problems should advance directives be made legally enforceable as is the case in some American states.

There is for instance the possibility that a patient could inadvertently misdirect the doctor by an inadequate appreciation of changed circumstances or of the evolution of new treatments in the unforeseeable future.

The Ethics Group of the Association for Palliative Medicine issued a Statement on Advance Directives in 1993:

Association for Palliative Medicine, Ethics Group – Statement on Advance Directives

The Association represents doctors working in hospices and with specialist palliative care teams. Our main areas of work are with patients suffering from advanced malignant disease, advanced neurodegenerative diseases and advanced immunodeficiency.

A prerequisite for the appropriate care of such patients is recognition of the fundamental importance of patient autonomy. This requires highly developed communication skills with a commitment to careful unhurried listening and frequent reassessment of patients' wishes. The principle of informed consent to treatment at all stages of advancing disease, therefore, underpins palliative care. As a contribution to this process we recognize potential value in the documented expression of patients' general views about medical care.

A comprehensive review of the subject of advance directives is given in the statement of November 1992 by the British Medical Association. The BMA is not in favour of legal enforcement of such documents, a view with which we entirely agree.

From our working practice we would highlight particularly the following points against advance directives being enforceable by law.

1   Ambiguity and scope for misinterpretation.
Whatever care is put into the wording of advance directives the precise meaning of terms such as terminal illness, active treatment and competence will always be open to doubt.
2   Pressure on vulnerable groups.
The likelihood of the elderly and chronic sick who feel themselves to be a burden being pressurised into signing advance directives will increase if such documents become legally binding.
3   Bias

Bias against active treatment inherent in some published advance directives may limit rather than enhance an individual's autonomy.

4   Implications for euthanasia.

We deplore moves to make advance directives legally binding as part of a gradualist policy to legalise euthanasia.

We believe that the interests of patients will be best served by resisting attempts to make advance directives enforceable by law.

References

[1] Maguire, P. and Faulkner, A. (1988) Communicate with Cancer Patients: Handling uncertainty, collusion and denial. *British Medical Journal*, **297**: 272–4.

[2] Stedeford, A. (1981) Couples Facing Death. *British Medical Journal*, **17**: 283.

[3] Neuberger, J. (1987) *Caring for Dying People of Different Faiths*. Lisa Sainsbury Foundation, London. Austen Cornish, London.

See also Further Reading, page 99.

2 | Control of Distressing Symptoms

Introduction

This chapter describes the control of the most common distressing symptoms which are found in terminal illness. Although the assessment and management of each symptom is described separately, many patients have several symptoms at the same time. Figure 2.1 shows those symptoms that occur most commonly in the last year of life, as reported by bereaved carers. All of these symptoms are discussed in this chapter.

Some key points relate to the management of all symptoms:

1   Ask the patient for their assessment of how much the symptom troubles them.
2   Identify the cause and remember that this may not be the cancer but could be a side effect of treatment or due to a previous or new illness.
3   Choose an appropriate treatment: as well as drugs, this could include surgery, radiotherapy, nerve blocks or chemotherapy.[2,3] The value of communication, information and emotional support should not be overlooked.
4   Prescribe appropriately, taking into account:
    (a) **site of action** eg non-steroidal anti-inflammatory drugs (NSAIDs) used to reduce the production of tissue-sensitizing prostaglandins, for instance, in bone pain
    (b) **duration of action** eg controlled release morphine 12 hourly, morphine 4 hourly
    (c) **dosage range** eg normal dose range very often extended, for example, in the use of laxatives
    (d) **symptom response** eg antidepressants can take up to 14 days, although when these are used as a co-analgesic a more rapid response is achieved
    (e) **side effects** eg for opioids, constipation
    (f) **interactions** eg dexamethasone and phenytoin; concomitant administration results in reduced effect of the corticosteroid. Drug regimens should be kept as simple as possible and be given orally whenever possible.
5   Consider psychosocial and spiritual factors.
6   Communicate and give information about both the cause of the symp-

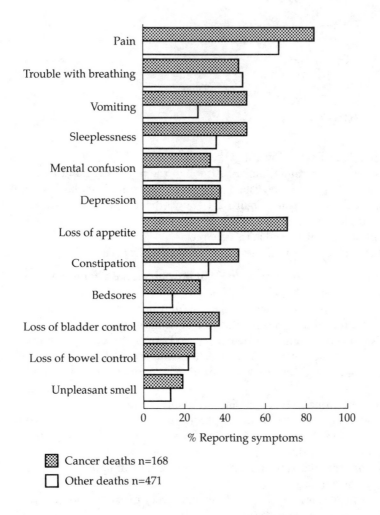

Figure 2.1: Symptoms in the last year of life, as reported by carers. (Drawn from data reported by Cartwright[1]).

toms and the plans for treatment, including how soon it is likely to take effect and any side effects which may occur or need to be addressed.

7 Examine and re-assess often. Monitor the response to treatment. Clinical audits of symptom control can improve care. There are now some tested and validated tools for the audit of palliative care, including the recording of symptoms. For example the Support Team Assessment Schedule, the

Edmonton Symptom Assessment Scale (both of which record several symptoms including pain)[4]

Pain

Pain is a complex and unpleasant sensory and emotional experience. A useful clinical definition is that the pain is of whatever severity the patient says it is. In terminal illness pain can be classified into four main groups, all of which require specific attention:

- physical
- emotional (anxiety, fears, depression)
- social (isolation, embarrassment)
- spiritual (desolation).

This list can also be regarded from a different standpoint. If someone has overwhelming *physical* pain, there are also emotional and mental consequences, such as an inability to concentrate or emotional exhaustion; social consequences (a patient may have no desire to talk and may say 'Go away and leave me alone'); spiritual consequences (a sense of despair and 'What have I done to deserve this?'). Just as the pathological condition is destroying the patient physically, so it may also as a consequence destroy the patient emotionally, socially and spiritually. Such chronic pain is not like the pain of a minor injury, nor does it have any protective or useful purpose. The priority is therefore to treat the pain rigorously and effectively.

Pain assessment

To establish the nature of the pain a full description should be obtained from the patient and their family, paying particular attention to its onset, character, severity, site, quality (what it is like), radiation, and provoking and relieving factors; and also its relationship to meals, movement, bowels, micturition and mood. A body chart (*see* Appendix 6), drawn with or by the patient, is a useful communication tool when assessing pain. The locations of different pains can be described and the features of the different pains can be identified. In advanced cancer it is common for patients to have two or more pains with different causes. An analgesic history is essential and this needs to include the analgesics being swallowed, information on analgesics tried, which were successful or not, doses, and any side effects. Monitoring pain control is essential for good management. The aim is to completely alleviate pain with as few side effects as possible.

Pain tolerance

A patient's pain tolerance may be lowered by fear, anger, isolation, loneliness, restlessness, exhaustion, and depression. Conversely it may be raised by rest and adequate sleep, sympathy, information, good communication, congenial surroundings, confidence in the carers, and, in some cases, diversion. A constant line of attack on pain therefore is to do everything possible to raise the pain tolerance.

Incidence of pain

A survey of bereaved carers indicated that 75% of cancer patients and 69% of other patients experienced pain in their last year of life[1]. Many patients will require opioids. In a survey at St Joseph's Hospice to find the proportion of patients in severe pain, 33% needed at least 30 mg of oral morphine four hourly at some time. A survey of cancer patients in the Bloomsbury home care team showed that 47% required slow release morphine, and most achieved good pain control until death taking between 30 mg and 60 mg twice daily[5]. These doses are generally considered to be modest: a few patients may require ten times this dose. Effective pain control is therefore a major challenge for those caring for terminally ill patients.

Common types of pain

Pain can be classified into that which is visceral, soft tissue, bone, nerve, secondary spasm (eg from the gut, bladder or rectum), or central nervous system pain. These different types of pain require different treatments and one patient may have several types of pain. Box 2.1 shows the common types of pains found in cancer and their treatment. Continuous pain due to soft tissue infiltration usually responds well to most analgesics and to morphine, but pain due to infiltration of the bone responds poorly to morphine and is usually controlled by radiotherapy or non-steroidal anti-inflammatory drugs (NSAIDs). Stabbing or burning pain due to nerve involvement responds poorly to morphine and usually needs tricyclics or anti-convulsants as well. NSAIDs, tricyclics and anti-convulsants used to assist pain control in this way are often referred to as adjuvant analgesics.

World Health Organization recommendations for pain control

This recommends that, for opioid responsive pains, analgesics should be administered:

- by the mouth (whenever possible this is optimal)
- by the clock (to allow pain to re-emerge before administering the next dose causes unnecessary suffering and encourages tolerance[6]. Drugs should be

Box 2.1: Common types of pains found in cancer and their treatment

Description of pain	Likely cause	Primary treatment	Also consider:
Continuous, severe	Visceral or soft tissue infiltration	Analgesics, eg if mild – paracetamol; if severe – morphine	Low-dose steroids, nerve block, if effective in reducing tumour; radiotherapy or chemotherapy may help
Made worse by movement, may be tender	Bone metastasis, if sudden onset consider pathological fracture	Radiotherapy, NSAID, consider pinning a fracture or bone at risk of fracture	Analgesics, eg morphine, nerve block, low-dose steroids; consider Transcutaneous Electric Nerve Stimulation (TENS)
'Stabbing, burning' or unpleasant sensory changes. Often severe	Nerve destruction or compression – neuropathic pain	Analgesics, eg morphine plus antidepressant or anti-convulsant	High-dose steroids; if compression, nerve block; consider TENS
'Comes and goes' related to bowels or to ureter	Colic, due to bowel obstruction, constipation or ureteric colic	Remove cause, if possible. Faecal softeners	Antispasmodics, analgesics. Obstruction: high-dose steroids or surgery
Headaches associated with nausea and vomiting, photophobia	Raised intracranial pressure	High-dose steroids. Raise head of bed. Carbamazepine.	NSAID, consider further radiotherapy
Continuous severe pain, occasionally 'throbbing' and not responding to opioids	Consider infection, especially in tumours of head and neck	Add broad spectrum antibiotic to regime	NSAID, drain abscess

given regularly and not as required. For morphine and codeine, except controlled release preparations, 4 hourly is optimal.
• by the ladder, *see* Figure 2.2.

Mild pain

This only needs mild analgesics such as:

• paracetamol tablets BP – 500 mg: 1 or 2, 4–6 hourly
• aspirin dispersable BP – 300 mg: 1 or 2, 4–6 hourly.

Paracetamol is useful in a variety of pains, including skeletal muscle pains and mild cancer-related pains. Doses of 1 g four hourly do not produce adverse effects, and there are no reports of liver toxicity with doses of 4–6 gms daily in divided doses in cancer patients[7]. Paracetamol also has an antipyretic effect: it will reduce fever. Aspirin is also effective in many patients but its disadvantage is its tendency to cause gastric irritation. Weak opioids have been recommended if mild pain persists[8]. This is the second step in the analgesic ladder.

Examples of weak opioids include:

• Co-codamol tablets (codeine phosphate 8 mg, paracetamol 500 mg), 1–2 tablets, 8 hourly
• Dihydrocodeine tablets BP – 30 mg, 1–2 tablets, 4 hourly
• Dextropropoxyphene capsules BP – equivalent of 65 mg HCI salt, 1–2 tablets, 4–8 hourly
• Dextropropoxyphene and paracetamol (co-proxamol – 32.5 mg dextropropoxyphene, 325 mg paracetamol, 2 tablets, 4–8 hourly).

Dihydrocodeine is approximately one tenth as potent as morphine and dextropropoxyphene approximately one sixth as potent. Dextropropox-

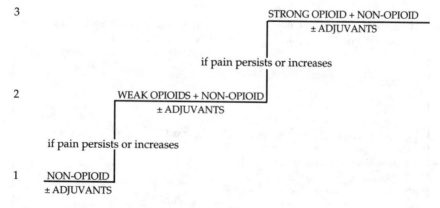

Figure 2.2: World Health Organization analgesic ladder[8]

yphene has a prolonged half life which can result in accumulation especially in those with poor renal functions.

Some experienced palliative practitioners will miss out the second step in the WHO ladder, moving directly to a low dose of a strong opioid if pain persists[5,9]. They argue that weak opioids have greater adverse effects.

Severe pain

As soon as it is apparent that these or similar mild analgesics are no longer effective there should be no hesitation in using strong opioids – the third step in the analgesic ladder.

Unfortunately these drugs are often withheld for fear of drowsiness, addiction or respiratory depression. This is inappropriate. Drowsiness, if it does occur, soon wears off. When opioid drugs are given regularly to control cancer pain, addiction and tolerance are rarely seen. Respiratory depression is rarely a problem: pain acts as the physiological antagonist to respiratory depression.

Guidelines for use of opioid drugs

These should be given in adequate strength earlier rather than later in the illness. Once the correct dose has been ascertained, they should be administered regularly and given in a form to ensure absorption. The dose should be monitored frequently and side effects, such as nausea and especially constipation, controlled[10].

Oral opioids

This is the route of choice. Morphine sulphate is the drug of choice, with extensive experience and research demonstrating its value in many types of pain. Morphine sulphate is available as a solution or as tablets which need to be given 4 hourly, and it is available in a controlled release formulation which can be given twice a day. Examples of morphine tablets and solutions are shown in Box 2.2.

Box 2.2: Examples of morphine preparations

Morphine elixir (eg oramorph oral solution) 2 mg/ml.

Morphine elixir, concentrated (eg oramorph concentrated oral solution) 20 mg/ml + calibrated dropper.

Instant-release morphine sulphate (eg sevredol tablets) available as 10 mg and 20 mg.

Controlled-release morphine sulphate (eg MST tablets, SRM-Rhotard tablets) available as 10 mg, 30 mg, 60 mg, 100 mg and 200 mg tablets – or in a suspension.

Diamorphine and hydromorphone (used widely in North America but not in Britain) are preferred by some doctors and it is important to remember that these are not equipotent with morphine. When dispensed as a liquid, diamorphine is reported to be less stable than morphine and tends to have a limited shelf life[11]. Some commercially available preparations of morphine include a preservative to extend shelf-life. Diamorphine and hydromorphone have a place in the subcutaneous delivery of opioids (see page 43).

Other opioids have no advantage over these strong opioids. Buprenorphine is a partial antagonist and should not be used at the same time as other opioids. Pethidine and dextromoramide and pentazocine have too short a half life and are unsuitable for treatment of severe pain, particularly cancer pain. Toxic metabolites have also been reported. To assist conversions, Appendix 4 shows the approximate oral morphine equivalent of various different drugs.

Establishing the dosage of opioids

The starting dose of opioids will depend on previous analgesic needs, on renal function, and on the severity of pain. If a patient is no longer experiencing pain relief from weak opioids, then a first prescription should be morphine solution orally 5 or 10 mg, every four hours depending on the patient's age, size and previous drug therapy. The dose of morphine has to be titrated against the patient's pain, and if there is breakthrough pain, the dose should be increased to 10 or 15 mg 4 hourly and thereafter in increments of 5 mg daily until the patient is pain free throughout 24 hours. That is then the correct dose for a patient's pain at that time. After 20 mg, 4 hourly daily increments are 10 mg, and after 100 mg 4 hourly daily increments are 20 mg.

When converting to controlled release morphine, the same 24 hour dose of morphine is given but it is now divided into two 12 hourly doses. For example, a 20 mg dose of oral morphine solution every four hours would equate to one 60 mg controlled release morphine tablet every 12 hours.

Rectal opioids

If oral medication is inappropriate because of vomiting, dysphagia, weakness or suspected malabsorption, rectal administration may be considered. Provided there is no rectal or pelvic pathology hindering insertion or absorption, the result can be almost as good as that of oral administration. The same doses as for oral medication should be used. Morphine suppositories are available in strengths of 10 mg, 15 mg, 20 mg, and 30 mg and these must be given 4 hourly. Oxycodone suppositories are also available on special order and only need to be given three times a day. Although not licensed for rectal use, oral controlled release morphine (MST) tablets have been given rectally to control pain[12, 13].

Parenteral opioids

If oral or rectal administration are not appropriate, the opioid has to be given by injection. Diamorphine is the drug of choice because its greater solubility enables larger doses to be given in a smaller volume of fluid. Small injection volumes are also possible with hydromorphone (used in the USA and Canada). The ratios for oral to parenteral conversion are as follows: 3 mg of oral morphine is equivalent to 1 mg of parenteral diamorphine or 0.2 mg parenteral hydromorphone or 1.5 mg of parenteral morphine (*see* Appendix 4).

The preferred parenteral route is subcutaneous. Small volume subcutaneous injections through a fine 25 g needle is kinder to patients and is as effective as an intramuscular injection. The intravenous route is usually avoided and tolerance has been described when diamorphine has been given by this route.

If 4 hourly injections are required, it is far better to use an infusion device such as a syringe driver (*see* Appendix 5). If not available, one may be borrowed from the local hospice, support team, Macmillan nurses or hospital. A 24 hour dose of diamorphine (an antiemetic may be added, if necessary) is drawn into a 10 ml syringe which is fitted into the driver to which a canula with a butterfly needle is attached. The setting is adjusted to deliver the contents of the syringe at a controlled rate, usually over 24 hours. The butterfly is inserted subcutaneously (usually in the anterior chest wall) avoiding any oedematous regions. Excellent and continuous pain control is achieved with this method and often with a smaller total dose of medication. The syringe is recharged daily and it is wise to change the site of the needle every two to three days. Occasionally local indurations develop at the needle site. These are usually caused not by morphine, but by other drugs added to control nausea, vomiting or other symptoms[14].

Intraspinal opioids

These are useful in a small proportion of patients who have severe unrelieved pain and for whom opioids are accompanied by unacceptable adverse effects. Sensory afferent fibres of peripheral nerves terminate in the dorsal horns of the spinal cord, where there are high concentrations of opioid receptors. Local action of opioids in this region suppresses the transmission of pain stimuli. Consequently, by placing small amounts of opioids in the epidural or intrathecal space, it is possible to achieve sustained pain control. This can be done by inserting a tunnelled epidural or intrathecal catheter, by implanting an intraspinal system, such as a Port-a-Cath system, or by implanting a fully computerized pump. The first two of these systems can be used to give bolus doses, continuous delivery, or continuous delivery and patient activated bolus doses. The most commonly used drugs are: morphine sulphate, which has a slow absorbency rate; diamorphine, which is very soluble and may be used in high concentrations; fentanyl and bupivacaine, which are especially helpful with difficult localized bone pain; and steroids, which can reduce peri-neurial oedema. Spinal routes need practitioners skilled in the technique of catheter placement and a nursing team which understands spinal catheter care[15].

Transdermal opioids

Fentanyl is available in North America and consists of patches delivering a range of rates over 72 hours. Transdermal fentanyl has the advantage of con-venient continuous administration and longer duration of action and there-fore may be preferred by some patients. It has been used effectively to control cancer pain and is currently being tested in the UK. It may be of use for patients in whom the parental route is undesirable because of coagulation dis-orders or severe immunosuppression. However, it may be costly and has a slow onset of action, slow titration, and slower reversal of side effects: more information is needed[16].

Inhaled opioids

Inhaled morphine is mainly of value in controlling dyspnoea (see page 50) and has been used to control post-operative pain. It is not suitable for patients with severe congestive failure or comatose states and requires further research in pain control[16].

Side effects of opioids

Nausea and vomiting occur initially in about a third of patients[12]. This is dose-related and tends to wear off in about a week, enabling antiemetics (if these have been required, see Box 2.4) to be reduced or withdrawn. Constipa-tion occurs in almost all patients taking opioids. Laxatives should be pre-scribed routinely for all patients taking opioids. Once established, constipation can be intractable and cause great distress (see Box 2.5). A dry mouth occurs in about 40% of patients but this can be treated with local mea-sures such as offering ice cubes, frozen fruit juice, pineapple chunks, or frozen tonic water, perhaps with a drop of gin, to suck. Sedation is thought to occur in up to 20% of patients, but again this is dose-related and is usually mild and self-limiting, ending in five to seven days. Sweating, dizziness, blurred vision, confusion, hallucinations, and myoclonus occur occasionally but usually only when doses have been very rapidly escalated. For an opioid overdose, naloxone 0.2–0.4 mg by intravenous injection should be given, and repeated as often as necessary. Naloxone is much shorter acting than most opioids.

Adjuvant analgesia

While opioids are the most useful drugs for controlling severe pain, there are other therapies, as shown in Box 2.1, which may be indicated for special types of pain, and which may be used in addition to, or as an adjunct to, opioids.

Bone pain

This usually arises from bone metastases from primary cancer of the lung, breast, prostate or thyroid, although other tumours may metastasize into bone; and, of course, primary malignancy may occur in bone as well. The pain is a dull, boring sensation, exacerbated by movement and pressure.

Radiotherapy is the most effective treatment as, apart from relieving pain, it can produce regression. Non-steroidal anti-inflammatory drugs (NSAIDs) act as anti-prostaglandins within the bone and are often very effective in relieving bone pain. There are seven different chemical classes of NSAIDs and patients who do not respond to NSAIDs in one class may respond to those in another. Generally, the more potent the drug the greater its side effects. Of the many drugs available, the most useful are: naproxen (250–500 mg twice daily), ibuprofen (400 mg three to four times per day, flurbiprofen (50–100 mg three times a day), diclofenac (25–50 mg tds) or indomethacin (25–50 mg tds).

Steroids can also relieve bone pain. A starting dose of dexamethasone 8 mg daily is usually required. Once pain relief is achieved the dose may be reduced gradually. There is data which suggests that the risk of a peptic ulcer is doubled in patients treated chronically with steroids, although this may be associated with the use of NSAIDs[17]. Therefore, if the patient is at risk of a peptic ulcer ranitidine 150 mg twice daily may be needed.

Biphosphonates inhibit osteoclastic function and are used to manage hypercalcaemia in advanced cancer. Their role in controlling bone pain and reducing the incidence of fracture is currently under review.

Immobilization is occasionally helpful and surgery is indicated where there is a high risk of fracture or if a bone has already fractured. Patients considered to be at risk should be referred for an orthopaedic opinion. Anaesthetic techniques may also have value in the control of bone pain.

Neuropathic pain

This is often a very severe pain associated with abnormal sensation including dysaesthesia (unpleasant, abnormal sensation), causalgia (sustained burning pain) or allodynia (pain due to a stimulus which does not normally provoke pain). The patient may describe pain in an area of abnormal sensation, for example, in a numb area, or may describe shooting or stabbing pains. Examination may reveal abnormal movement or reflexes but this is often not found. Neuropathic pains can be caused by compression or invasion of the primary tumour or metastases; they may be indirectly related to the cancer, such as a herpetic neuralgia, or they may be occasionally as a result of chemotherapy, radiotherapy, or post surgery.

Opioids are typically not very effective in the control of neuropathic pains. Of benefit is the addition of tricyclic antidepressants, such as amitriptyline (25 mg starting dose, increasing gradually to 100 mg), imipramine and clomipramine. Their action is independent of their effects on mood and may be of particular benefit for 'burning' pain. The drug takes some time to have an effect, and, though some relief may be found in under one week, a trial of six weeks increasing the dose, is usually recommended before a drug is thought not to be effective.

Anticonvulsants, such as carbamazepine (100 mg at night, increasing if necessary up to 400 mg, 12 hourly), sodium valproate (starting dose 200 mg twice daily, increasing as necessary to 400 mg tds), phenytoin, flecainide (100 mg, 12 hourly) and clonazepam have all been used with success, particularly for shooting or stabbing pains. As with antidepressants, the dose is increased slowly and a response may be seen within a week.

Local anaesthetic agents, such as lignocaine, have been reported with success for cancer patients with neuropathic pain which has not responded to systemic or spinal opioids. Dexamethasone (16–24 mg daily and avoiding a dose after 6.00 pm) has also been of use, particularly for patients who have a degree of nerve compression. The dose should be reduced to the lowest which will control the symptoms. In some cases a nerve block is considered[18].

Transcutaneous Electric Nerve Stimulation (TENS)

The gate theory of pain suggests that stimulation of large afferent nerve fibres reduces the input from peripheral pain receptors to the brain. It is also postulated that endogenous opioids produced by TENS assist analgesia. TENS is produced from a portable, battery-powered stimulator and applied through small electrodes on the skin. The results are variable but it has been used for many types of pain and has virtually no adverse effects[19]. It has been suggested that continuous stimulation is best for pains due to tissue damage, such as bone metastases, joint pain, or visceral pain, and pulsed acupuncture-like stimulation is better for neuropathic pain[9,19]. Optimum siting of the electrodes and adjustment of the stimulator may not be obtained at once and there is scope for trial with the help of the patient to obtain the best result.

Case history

Four years ago when Mr P. retired, he and his wife went to live in a warmer country. They were enjoying their retirement until nine months ago, when Mrs P. began to complain of low back and deep pelvic pains. The local doctor treated this as a musculoskeletal condition and arranged for physiotherapy. However, exercises exacerbated the discomfort which gradually became more disabling. After six months, with no sign of improvement, they returned to London for further advice. X-rays revealed scattered metastases in the lumbo-sacral spine and right side of the pelvis, and biopsy confirmed that these were malignant deposits from an unidentified primary. Radiotherapy gave some relief but after three months, during which she developed weakness of her right leg, she was admitted to St Joseph's Hospice. On admission she was in excruciating pain in the right pelvis, exacerbated even by the slightest movement. There was local bone tenderness and also severe neuritic pain radiating to the right ankle. She had been taking controlled release morphine 10 mg bd with no relief. She also had retention of urine, with a distended bladder and a flaccid paresis of the right leg. She was treated with oral morphine which was rapidly increased in dosage over the first four days to 40 mg 4 hourly. She was also given NSAID treatment in the form of flurbiprofen 100 mg tds, dexamethasone 12 mg daily, and a catheter was inserted. There was significant but inadequate pain relief from this treatment. Accordingly, an intrathecal nerve block was performed. This procedure gave her complete relief and she remained pain-free in the three months after it was performed. The doses of morphine and dexamethasone were reduced. She was up in a chair for most of the day, busy with various handicrafts and completely relaxed, although her general condition slowly weakened and she died peacefully with no recurrence of pain.

Muscle spasm

This can be extremely painful. The treatment can include: physiotherapy plus baclofen (5 mg, 8 hourly titrating slowly) or a benzodiazepine, such as diazepam. The latter may cause unacceptable drowsiness and doses can range from 2 mg to 5 mg tds, possibly with 10 mg at night. Nocturnal cramps are occasionally helped by quinine sulphate (300 mg at night) and peripheral spasms may be helped by nerve blocks.

Colic or smooth muscle spasm pain

This can be due to partial obstruction in the intestine, urinary tract or biliary tract. Any cause, such as constipation, needs to be treated, see Box 2.1, but antispasmodics such as hyoscine hydrobromide, sublingually or hyoscine butylbromide (10–20 mg, four times a day or 30–180 mg subcutaneous infusion per 24 hours) can be helpful (see also page 55, Box 2.4). Continued use may produce troublesome side effects such as drowsiness, dry mouth, blurred vision or urinary retention.

Raised intracranial pressure

This causes severe headache, neck stiffness and vomiting as well as neurological defects (see Box 2.1).
    If the symptoms are due to intracranial malignancy, a trial of high dose steroids is well worthwhile. Steroids are believed to increase cerebral blood flow but reduce blood volume and so reverse ischaemia and intracranial pressure.

Dexamethasone may be used as a therapeutic trial in a dose of 16–24 mg daily (although experienced palliative practitioners have tested doses as high as 96 mg per day). Any response will be evident within a few days and if there is no response within six days the dexamethasone should be discontinued. If it is used for a longer period, withdrawal should be gradual.

If there is a response (and the response is occasionally dramatic), the dexamethasone should be continued, although the dose will have to be reduced gradually otherwise adverse effects including Cushingoid features will develop. The reduction of dosage will have to be empirical, and the level of dose will depend on balancing the benefit against any side effects from the dexamethasone.

When patients are on continual high doses of dexamethasone, oral candidias (thrush) and other fungal infections are common, especially in frail patients (*see* page 62 for treatment). Regular testing for glycosuria or hyperglycaemia is advisable. Gastric irritation and peptic ulceration are suspected to occur more commonly, but the evidence is unclear. If ulceration is suspected, or a patient is believed to be at risk, or on NSAIDs as well, ranititide 150 mg twice daily may be given.

As the tumour continues to increase in size, the symptoms of raised intracranial pressure will usually return despite the steroid. When this happens the symptoms should be treated by analgesics and antiemetics. In general the NSAIDs are more useful than opioids. Many patients with intracranial tumours will require treatment with anticonvulsants, and it is important to note that anticonvulsants will reduce the effectiveness of dexamethasone.

Infection and ulceration

Cellulitis and abscesses should be treated with appropriate antibiotics and drainage, if necessary. Sores, ulcers and fungating lesions can be extremely painful. If the tumour responds to chemotherapy, this may help these lesions but the side effects of the chemotherapy must be weighed against the severity of the problem for the patient. Short acting opioids or inhalation of nitrous oxide and oxygen before a drainage procedure or dressing may also be helpful.

Other causes of pain

A dying patient may suffer great distress from conditions unrelated to the terminal disease, such as toothache, musculoskeletal conditions, thrombophlebitis, constipation, haemorrhoids, and various infections. They should respond to specific treatment, and such treatment should not be withheld because the patient is dying.

Case history

Mr S. was a 69-year-old widower, who had been diagnosed as having an extensive squamous cell cancer of the lung three months previously. The cancer was inoperable and he was short of breath after walking to the toilet. He lived alone, had been a smoker since his teens, and had two caring children, both now married. On being told his diagnosis he expected to die quite quickly and decided that he would prefer to be in a hospice. After admission his chest pain and dyspnoea were reasonably well-controlled with a small dose of opioids. However, his main problem was night pain due to an ischaemic foot. This had troubled him for several years but he had not been thought suitable for an operation because his continuing to smoke would have given him no long-term benefit. However this pain was now worse and given his shortened life expectancy, we arranged for him to be seen by an anaesthetist, who assessed him and treated him with a lumbar sympathetic nerve block. He achieved a dramatic response to this and the foot pain went completely, giving him the best nights of sleep he had had for years and a much improved quality of life during his remaining four months, until he died from his lung cancer.

Respiratory Symptoms

Dyspnoea

Definitions and incidence

Dyspnoea is distressing difficulty in breathing. It is found in just over 50% of patients in the last year of life but becomes more common as death approaches. Patients are particularly prone to dyspnoea if they have primary or secondary cancer in the lung[20] or chronic obstructive airways disease or asthma. Patients with dyspnoea have been shown to have a shortened survival compared to those who do not[21].

Assessment

To establish the nature of dyspnoea a full description should be obtained from the patient and from the family, paying particular attention to its onset, timing, severity, associated symptoms (eg wheeze or cough) and exacerbating and relieving factors. There are numerous causes and often several co-exist. Common causes are shown in Box 2.3.

Box 2.3: Common causes of dyspnoea in terminal illness

> *Mechanical factors – disease within the lung,* eg primary or secondary tumour, mesothelioma, lymphangitis carcinomatosis, lung collapse or consolidation, infection, emphysema, chronic obstructive airways disease, asthma, bronchospasm, fibrosis post radiotherapy; *disease outside the lung,* eg pleural effusion, ascites, hepatomegaly, mediastinal or paratracheal lymphadenopathy, superior vena cava obstruction, pericardial effusion.
> *Impaired diffusion of respiratory gases* – eg pulmonary embolism, pulmonary oedema, ischemic heart disease.
> *Biochemical factors* – anaemia, uraemia.
> *Psychogenic factors* – anxiety, fear, depression, hyperventilation syndrome (characteristics are dyspnoea plus tingling or muscle tremors, faintness, dizziness, and sometimes sweating, palpitations and angina).

Treatment

If the patient is severely hypoxic, they will require oxygen, 100% via a face mask, if they have no history of respiratory problems, and 24% via a Venturi mask, if they have or had previous chronic obstructive airways disease with carbon dioxide retention[22,23]. If a patient is not hypoxic but complaining of dyspnoea, immediate measures to provide some relief include increasing air movement over the patient's face with a fan or open window. Ice placed in front of the fan will provide a cool blast of air. Explanation, massage, sitting upright and distraction may also help.

Other treatment measures will depend on the cause and clearly ventricular failure, infection, superior vena cava or tracheal obstruction, and asthma require appropriate treatment.

The main options for treating dyspnoea in terminal illness include the following[22-25]:

- Bronchodilators – usually given in nebulized or inhaler form. Of most benefit for air flow obstruction, although there is some evidence that it helps patients to increase lung volume even when air flow obstruction is not apparent.
- Opioids – in small doses these cause subjective release of dyspnoea and may also help to reduce anxiety, stop pain from lung disease such as pleurisy and improve heart failure. Nebulized morphine may reduce dyspnoea due to lung pathology, such as lymphangitis. A starting dose of 5 mg, 4 hourly is common.
- Steroids – relieve bronchospasm and oedema around lung or mediastinal cancers and lymphangitis carcinomatosis (recommended doses range from 8–24 mg dexamethasone daily, reducing to the lowest dose that controls symptoms). Dexamethasone should be given immediately for tracheal or superior vena cava obstruction.
- Antibiotics – are helpful in relieving dyspnoea due to pneumonia. They are particularly useful if symptoms of pneumonia are hampering the quality of

life and if cough or fever is a problem. They would not be indicated if they prolonged a patient's dying but did not improve quality of life.

- Oxygen – is important for severely hypoxic patients. If it is used in the home, strategic siting of oxygen, for example, in a place where the patient normally develops dyspnoea, may improve quality of life and mobility. Oxygen at home needs careful planning: the introduction of an oxygen cylinder or an oxygen concentrator can be distressing, especially in the last days of life, and at this very late stage may be of little benefit.

- Physiotherapy – coughing exercises, postural drainage, humidified air, percussion vibrations and forced expiration may help to clear bronchial secretions. Obviously these should not be too tiring for the patient. Breathing exercises to teach the patient slow diaphragmatic breathing rather than fast thoracic breathing helps the uptake of oxygen and the excretion of carbon dioxide, which occurs more effectively at the bases of the lungs rather than at the apices. In home care family members can be taught massage by the physiotherapist.

- Atropinics – hyoscine hydrobromide and hyoscine butylbromide will reduce excessive bronchial secretions and are useful in treating noisy secretions (death rattle) in an unconscious patient. It should be remembered, however, that these secretions are often more distressing to the relatives who hear them than to the patient. Both drugs are sedating and it may not be appropriate to entirely eliminate the noise due to excess secretions. The dose of hyoscine hydrobromide is 0.4 to 2.4 mg over 24 hours subcutaneously.

- Psychotropic drugs – these may relieve anxiety associated with dyspnoea but doses need to be small because of drowsiness. Diazepam (2–5 mg, three times a day) is sometimes helpful. Alcohol is also of value.

- Local anaesthetic inhalations – may be useful as second line treatment and probably work by blocking nerve receptors in the lung and also possibly causing bronchodilation. Particle diameter must be small enough to reach the alveoli and therefore jet or ultrasonic nebulizers are required. Bupivacaine (doses have been between 0.25–5%, inhaling 5 ml, 4 hourly) is used in preference to lignocaine, which works equally well but tastes unpleasant.

- Helium and oxygen (80% plus 20%) – are rarely used but may help dyspnoea due to malignant tracheal stenosis because the mixture is less dense than air and reduces the work of breathing.

- Prostaglandin inhibitors – remains to be evaluated but there is evidence that indomethacin reduces breathlessness in volunteers.

- Palliative procedures, such as radiotherapy and chemotherapy, are useful if the tumour is sensitive to these procedures; laser therapy or silicone or expandable metal stents may be used to relieve obstructing bronchial or tracheal tumours; and pleural taps may be used to drain plural effusions. Blood transfusions may sometimes help dyspnoea due to anaemia but not always. The risks and benefits for the patients and family for all these procedures must be carefully considered before they are carried out.

The hyperventilation provocation test may identify patients with hyperventilation syndrome. This test asks a patient to hyperventilate to see if this reproduces the symptoms of which they complain – twenty deep breaths is usually enough. Relief of symptoms by re-breathing into a paper bag is both therapeutic and diagnostic.

Cough

This can be caused by external irritants such as fumes, dust, smoke, air quality (very cold, hot or dry); inflammation (tumour infiltration or a respiratory infection anywhere along the respiratory tract – laryngitis, bronchitis, pneumonia); bronchospasm; seepage of fluid from lesions in the nose, mouth, or pharynx; irritation of the left recurrent laryngeal nerve by tumour and pulmonary oedema[24,25].

Many patients request a cough linctus but this is not particularly effective. Many therapies for cough will be the same as for dyspnoea (*see* page 49). In addition sips of hot drinks such as orange or blackcurrant juice are very soothing. Steam inhalations, with or without the addition of benzoin tincture or menthol and eucalyptus, can be effective especially when phlegm is thick. Bronchodilators and inhalation of a local anaesthetic may also be helpful.

If a cough suppressant is required, codeine linctus is very suitable. Opioids, which may be given to control pain or dyspnoea, also help to diminish cough and there is no need to prescribe both codeine linctus and morphine to suppress a cough. A small dose of morphine may be prescribed specifically for cough.

Ephedrine and medications containing it should be avoided due to the risk of urinary retention. A productive cough with mucopurulent sputum may be relieved by prescribing a broad spectrum antibiotic for a few days such as chloramphenicol (250–500 mg, orally, four times per day) or amoxycillin (250–500 mg, three times a day).

The frothy expectoration of pulmonary oedema is helped by diuretics such as frusemide (40 mg twice a day) or, if acute, by injection.

Most patients with persistent cough feel more comfortable when propped up and, as for dyspnoea, physiotherapy may be helpful.

Gastrointestinal Symptoms

Nausea and vomiting

There are many causes of nausea and vomiting, and the patient may feel ill and weak with dizziness, headaches and sweating. Causes include drugs (such as opioids, digoxin, cytotoxins, NSAIDs, steroids, oestrogens); radiotherapy; biochemical causes (such as, hypercalcaemia – *see* page 68 – and uraemia); infections (such as a urinary tract infection); gastric irritation; gastric outflow obstruction; intestinal obstruction; severe constipation; raised intracranial pressure; vestibular disturbance; coughing; and fear and anxiety[26,27].

Drugs suspected of causing nausea or vomiting should be withdrawn, if possible. If they are essential, they should be given in a form to diminish their nauseating propensity, for example, aspirin and prednisolone can both be given with an enteric coating.

Gastric irritation

Dyspepsia can be relieved by aluminium- and magnesium-containing antacids, such as gaviscon tablets to chew, or liquid 10 ml after meals and at bedtime, or asilone or diovol suspension, 5–10 ml before meals and at bedtime. If dyspepsia is severe drugs which reduce excess gastric acid secretion may help eg cimetidine (200 mg, three times a day) or ranitidine or omeprazol.

Oesophageal reflux

Suitable preparations are mucaine suspension, 5–10 ml, 15 minutes before meals and at bedtime or algicon tablets or suspension or medication suitable for gastric irritation. Omeprazole (20–40 mg daily for four weeks), cimetidine (200 mg, three times a day) or ranitidine (300 mg at night) also relieve symptoms. Gastric and duodenal ulcers should be treated with these drugs.

Gastric outflow obstruction and squashed stomach syndrome

This occurs in hepatomegaly or where there is a large abdominal tumour. It may also occur in carcinoma of the stomach (especially linitis plastica). There is a constant sensation of fullness and nausea with an oesophageal reflux and heartburn. Avoid large or heavy meals, which the patient will not want anyway. Give small amounts of fluid and bland foods frequently. Antacids and metoclopramide are helpful.

Vomiting from cerebral causes

Dexamethasone should be used as for raised intracranial pressure, (see page 47). This treatment reduces intracranial pressure but the improvement may only last for a few weeks (occasionally several months in slow growing tumours) as the tumour itself continues to grow. Remission of symptoms resulting from the administration of dexamethasone is only temporary, and when the symptoms return there is little purpose in continuing the dexamethasone.

Fear and anxiety

If emotional tension is thought to be a cause of nausea and vomiting then the patient's and their family's fears and concerns should be discussed. For management *see* pages 73–4.

Intestinal obstruction

Surgery may be considered in appropriate cases, for example, if it is thought that the patient may have several months to live, is willing to undergo an operation and medical and nursing colleagues agree there is a chance of improvement. However, in terminal illness it is usually inappropriate – patients may be too ill for an operation, and may have had surgery already and are now unlikely to benefit.

Many patients with inoperable malignant obstruction can be treated symptomatically. Pain and nausea are treated by analgesic and antiemetic drugs which may be given per rectum or by injection. If injections are needed regularly, the drugs may be given subcutaneously via a syringe driver. Some patients may continue to vomit once or twice a day but their pain and constant nausea can be relieved by appropriate medication.

The gastrokinetic antiemetics, such as metoclopramide and domperidone, should not be used for vomiting caused by intestinal obstruction. Hyoscine butylbromide is useful for both intestinal colic and vomiting of intestinal obstruction. It may be given as a single injection of 20 mg, included with other medications in the syringe driver in a daily dose of about 40 mg (up to 80 mg) or given orally 60–200 mg/day. Hyoscine hydrobromide can also be used. Patients often have continuous pain which requires treatment with morphine.

Nasogastric tubes and intravenous fluids are nearly always unnecessary but it is important to maintain mouth care and moisturize mucous membranes (*see* page 61).

Antiemetics

Suggested antiemetics are shown in Box 2.4. A small proportion of patients will require two antiemetics which have different main sites of action. Dexamethasone may be used as a second line treatment: it may potentiate other antiemetics and may help to reduce oedema in some cases of intestinal obstruction.

Constipation

This is a frequent concomitant of terminal illness. Impacted faeces may simulate abdominal malignancy. Once this impaction is relieved and bowel mobility restored, the patient's condition frequently improves dramatically.

Causes include inactivity, weakness, dehydration, diminished food intake, low fibre diet or direct effects from cancer such as narrowing of the gut, hypercalcaemia or nerve damage. Constipation may also result as a side effect of medication, such as opioids, iron, anticonvulsants, diuretics, vincristine or antimuscarinics, such as hyoscine.

Assessment is needed to clarify the changes in bowel habit, stool characteristics and abdominal and rectal examination.

A flow chart describing the main options for management is shown in

Box 2.4: Suggested antiemetics

Name	Main site of action	Daily dose	Routes	Notes
Cyclizine	Vomiting centre	100–200 mg	Oral, subcutaneous	First line treatment. Antihistamine, causes some drowsiness, dry mouth. May crystallize in syringe driver mixture.
Haloperidol	Chemoreceptor trigger zone	1.5–15 mg	Oral, subcutaneous	First line treatment. Wide variety of presentations including drops. High doses can cause extra-pyramidal effects
Metoclopramide	Upper gut, chemoreceptor trigger zone	30–100 mg	Oral, parenteral	Not advised in gastrointestinal obstruction
Domperidone	Upper gut, chemoreceptor trigger zone	30–180 mg	Oral, rectal	Not advised in gastrointestinal obstruction
Methotrimeprazine	Chemoreceptor trigger zone	50–200 mg	Oral, parenteral	Useful in intractable vomiting. Causes drowsiness, skin irritation when given subcutaneously.
Hyoscine hydrobromide	Vomiting centre	0.4–2.4 mg	Oral, parenteral, transdermal patches	Causes drowsiness, blurred vision, sometimes difficulty with micturition. Reduces noisy breathing, see page 51. Like hyoscine butylbromide it is useful in intestinal obstruction.

If one drug is not effective, a combination of drugs from different groups can be used. It may be necessary to administer antiemetics via a syringe driver for persistent vomiting.

Box 2.5. If intestinal obstruction is a possibility, only laxatives with a predominantly softening action, for example, docusate sodium or lactulose, should be used in order not to cause colic[28]. Otherwise in terminal illness a large dose of laxatives is usually needed. The bulk stimulants are less frequently used because patients are often unable to take copious fluid. It does help, however, if the patient can be persuaded to take extra fluid, particularly fruit drinks.

Diarrhoea

This is less common than constipation in terminal illness, except for patients who have HIV or AIDS (*see* Chapter 3 for diagnosis and treatment) or malabsorption.

Causes include drugs, such as some antibiotics, antacids, NSAIDs, laxatives, malabsorption from pancreatic tumours or bowel resection, obstruction from tumours or faecal impaction, radiotherapy, infection in the intestinal tract (especially in patients with HIV or AIDS), or anxiety and nervous tension. Spurious diarrhoea due to faecal impaction needs to be treated as for constipation.

Drug treatment is by loperamide (2 mg after each loose stool, up to 16 mg daily – experienced practitioners go up to 32 mg daily) available in capsules and syrup. Co-phenotrope (diphenoxylate and atropine sulphate, 100 parts to 1 part), or codeine phosphate (10–60 mg, 4 hourly) are alternatives. Morphine given to control pain will also help diarrhoea.

Steroid retention enemas are very useful for persistent diarrhoea caused by radiotherapy or tumour infiltration. Examples of these include Predsol, or Predenema or Colifoam. Oral aspirin may also help. Bulky offensive stools of steatorrhoea associated with pancreatic tumours require pancreatic supplements such as Pancrex V (pancreatin/protease/lipase and amylase) available as capsules or tablets and given with food.

Diarrhoea is occasionally due to fear or anxiety and these problems should be discussed and may also be helped by mild tranquillizers, such as diazepam, 2 mg, three times a day.

Dysphagia

This condition is caused by sore and dry mouth, pharyngeal obstruction, oesophageal obstruction (due to tumour, ulceration or stricture), neuromuscular disease (as may occur in motor neurone disease), central neurological failure (as in bulbar palsy) and fungal and other ulcerative conditions of the pharynx and oesophagus.

Treatment includes:

- maintain oral hygiene and moisturize the mouth
- treat any fungal infection, as this may have spread down the oesophagus, using nystatin oral suspension or if necessary a systemic anti-fungal antibiotic[29]

Box 2.5: Treatment of constipation

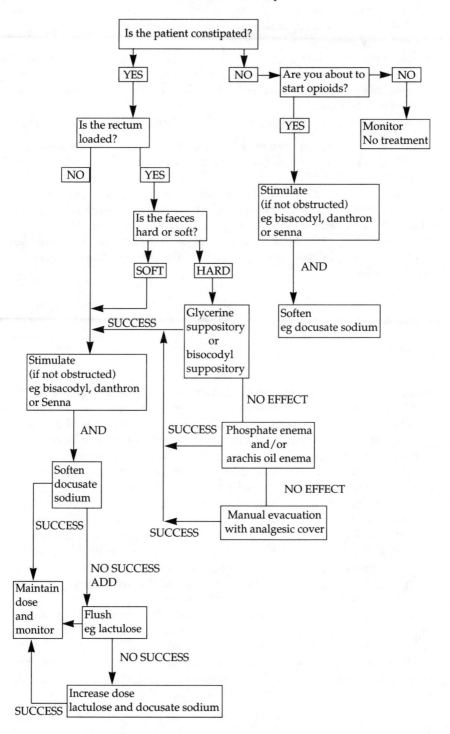

- provide food as the patient likes (small frequent meals, moist soft or puréed foods are often easier to eat)
- if the patient experiences problems when tipping the head backwards to drink, use a glass or cup which is full or nearly full – a picnic mug with a cut out for the nose may be helpful[30]
- dexamethasone, 4–16 mg daily, may improve dysphagia due to pharyngeal or oesophageal obstruction and will improve appetite
- consider the insertion of an oesophageal tube, which even in advanced cases may be helpful
- laser treatment or radiotherapy may reduce dysphagia caused by cancers.

Nutrition may be maintained via a fine bore nasogastric tube or endoscopic percutaneous gastronomy for patients with a prognosis of months rather than days.

To relieve distressing dehydration in patients with neuromuscular dysphagia, or for total organic dysphagia when the patient's condition is not terminal, a subcutaneous or intravenous infusion may be needed (*see* Dehydration page 69). In all cases control of pain and symptoms must be maintained and, if drugs cannot be given orally, parenteral or rectal routes will be needed.

Hiccup

This can be a very persistent and an annoying complaint. It is caused by diaphragmatic spasms due to gastric or abdominal distention, liver enlargement, diaphragmatic irritation from tumour infiltration, phrenic nerve irritation, vagus or thoracic nerve irritation, brain tumour or other causes of irritation in the central nervous system, and metabolic disorders such as uraemia[29].

For treatment, keep the patient propped up, give frequent small drinks and peppermint sweets to suck or peppermint water or oil (this facilitates belching). Gastric distention may be helped by small frequent meals, an antacid (such as asilone, 5–10 ml, four times daily), metoclopramide 10 ml, four times daily, which hastens gastric emptying. If hiccups are severe, try chlorpromazine 25 mg orally or IM (but it will cause drowsiness). An anticonvulsant, such as phenytoin 100 mg or sodium valproate, may help if a cerebral cause is suspected. Baclofen (5 or 10 mg twice daily), nifedipine (10–20 mg every eight hours) are worth trying for intractable hiccup[29, 31]. In severe cases consider whether radiotherapy or chemotherapy to reduce the size of the tumour may be helpful. Likewise consider steroids, although large doses are needed (for example, dexamethasone 16 mg daily). The dose should be reduced slowly as soon as a response is obtained.

Many patients also want to try folk remedies which often involve pharyngeal stimulation – such as drinking from the wrong side of a cup, crushed ice, a shock – and sometimes these can be helpful[29,32].

Anorexia

This is a common complaint of patients with advanced disease. Its causes include drugs, for example, cytotoxics, nausea and vomiting and fear of vomiting, gastrointestinal abnormalities or constipation, jaundice, biochemical changes such as uraemia or hypercalcaemia, anxiety and depression and sore or dry mouth. Through their effect of hastening gastric emptying, metoclopramide and domperidone (*see* page 55) may help to improve appetite.

The various tonics which have been prescribed have little effect. The most useful drugs are corticosteroids. Prednisolone (preferably enteric coated) 30 mg daily often produces a significant increase in appetite and the feeling of increased strength and well-being. Efficient mouth care is essential to eradicate soreness, especially due to thrush, and dryness. Small doses of antidepressants drugs may alleviate the patient's mood and increase appetite but antidepressants do not produce significant improvement in less than ten days (*see* Depression page 74). Small doses of anxiolytic drugs, for example, diazepam, may help anxiety.

Meals should be attractively presented in small quantities, and prepared in accordance with the patient's taste. An alcoholic aperitif is often helpful.

Cachexia

Cachexia (progressive weight loss, muscle weakness and emaciation) of terminal illness produces weakness and tiredness, which is very frustrating. The patient usually wants to maintain as much independence as possible, and may become depressed or angry when weakness prevents this.

Cachexia can occur despite reasonable food intake and is different from starvation[33,34]. Although the exact cause is not known, it has been associated with the release of tumour necrosis factors in cancer patients, infection, repeated tapping of pleural effusions or ascites, gastrointestinal obstruction, organ failure, nutritional deficiency or anaemia, anorexia, impaired digestion and absorption or increased energy expenditure due to catabolism from the cancer. All cancers can cause cachexia but it is more common in cancers of the pancreas and gastro-intestinal tract than in carcinomas of the breast or skin[33,35]. Weakness and fatigue without muscle wasting may also be caused by drugs (for example, diazepam, antidepressants or opioids), hypercalcaemia, septicemia, loss of sleep, anxiety and electrolyte disturbances such as hypo- or hyperglycaemia (this may be due to steroids, *see* pages 65–6)[36].

Management includes:

- explanation to the patient and family that it is not due to poor diet and that intensive feeding is only likely to make the patient uncomfortable, and will not prolong life
- dietary advice, as for anorexia. Oral nutrition should be attempted whenever appropriate, offering enjoyable food, attractively presented. Selected patients in whom oral nutrition is not possible may benefit from enteral nu-

trition, providing they have a prognosis of months or years rather than weeks. Parenteral nutrition has shown no significant benefits in terms of improving survival or comfort and is hardly ever indicated

- ensuring that the patient has everything they need close at hand and is resting more frequently, and providing them with gentle and unrushed nursing care and assistance with gentle mobilization and help with hygiene needs. Over zealous activity or numerous visitors may be exhausting.

Corticosteroids (prednisolone 30 mg or dexamethasone 4–8 mg in the morning) have sometimes been used, and are of particular benefit if they also help other symptoms such as dyspnoea, anorexia, nausea, and pain. Prolonged use should be avoided for cachexia because this can produce proximal myopathy, which exacerbates the weakness. High dose progestogens, eg megestrol acetate (160–480 mg daily) will be useful, again mainly by stimulating appetite, if the patient is expected to live for weeks or months[37-39].

Skin and Mouth Problems

Pressure sores

These develop through four stages – hyperaemia, blistering, broken skin, and penetration. Patients in terminal illness are at great risk of developing pressure sores, particularly if mobility is limited and diet and fluid intake is poor. Predisposing factors and the current state of a patient's pressure areas should be noted during the initial assessment, and an assessment scale, such as the Norton Scale (which has five headings – physical condition, mental state, activity, mobility and incontinence[40]) may help to determine those patients at risk.

Pressure sores can be prevented. The patient should be assisted to change position frequently. If this is not possible or appropriate, the following aids are helpful:

- special mattresses, which spread pressure more evenly over the body, for example, a spenco fibre mattress, an airwave mattress, a foam mattress (Pro-pad)
- special cushions, for example, Spenco and Roho
- heel and elbow pads and fleeces, such as sheepskin rugs and bootees
- bed cradles to prevent bed clothes from pressing down on the skin
- specialized beds, such as the Mediscus or Clinitron (these are expensive).

Any red or grazed areas may be protected using a vapour-permeable adhesive film dressing (eg Opsite or Tegaderm). Superficial sores may benefit from hydrocolloid dressings such as granuflex or tegasorb, which provide a moist healing environment. Foam and calcium alginate fibre are alternatives. Slough should be removed because it inhibits healing. Hydrogel dressings (eg

Intrasite) will benefit deeper or sloughy wounds and desloughing agents (eg Aserbine, streptokinase or hydrogen peroxide) may be used as second line treatment. Deeper cavities may need to be packed loosely with tulle dressings or silastic foam plugs to allow granulation.

When infections and/or cellulitis are present, take a swab for sensitivity and give the appropriate antibiotics systemically. Metronidazole (400 mg, three times daily) for anaerobic infections and flucloxacillin (250 mg, four times daily) for staphylococci are commonly required. Topical metronidazole gel (0.8%) may be used to control smell; otherwise topical antibiotics are not effective.

Pressure sores can be very painful; NSAIDs can often help to relieve this. Topical local anaesthetics may be helpful and light anaesthesia such as from nitrous oxide and oxygen via Entonox or analgesia from a short-acting opioid may be needed when applying dressings (*see* also Pain, page 37).

Fungating lesions

These are very distressing and the patient needs to be treated sensitively. The lesion should be cleaned daily with normal saline and either povidone iodine (Betadine) soaks, metronidazole gel or Jelonet applied. Persistent bleeding may be treated with gauze soaked in adrenaline (1:1000) applied for a few minutes; calcium alginate dressings reduce the likelihood of bleeding (*see* also Haemorrhage, page 69).

Some lesions will respond dramatically to hormone therapy, for example, in breast cancer, chemotherapy or radiotherapy, and this should be considered. If a response is achieved, the wound usually becomes dry and a simple non-adhesive dressing will suffice. If lesions are infected, a swab should be taken for culture and sensitivity and systemic antibiotics will be required. Metronidazole gel (400 mg, three times daily) is useful to control a foul smelling discharge due to anaerobic infections, often prevalent in deep sores and fistulae. Metronidazole is probably most effective when given orally.

Pain should be treated as for pressure sores (above). Comfort is the primary aim of treatment and although some healing is possible, significant improvement of extensive or necrotic lesions is often not possible.

Sore and dry mouth

This can be caused by fungal infections (thrush), dental problems (such as ill-fitting dentures, decaying teeth or a dental abscess), drugs (such as opioids, phenothiazines, antihistamines, tricyclic antidepressants), local radiotherapy, dehydration, malnutrition, immunosuppression, vitamin deficiency, herpes, blood dyscrasias, diabetes, aphthous ulceration, mouth breathing, cancrum oris, and debility reducing a person's ability to mouth care.

Routine mouth care is an essential procedure in terminal illness. To clean the mouth a soft-bristled, small-headed toothbrush with tap water and tooth paste is simple and refreshing, but a heavily coated tongue may require either vitamin C, ¼ of a 1 g effervescent tablet dissolved on the tongue four times a day, or mouthwashes of compound thymol glycerine, compound sodium chloride, hydrogen peroxide, sodium perborate, chlorhexidine or hexetidine[41,42].

Fungal infection

This is common and, if not treated, it may become regional or systemic in immunosuppressed patients[43,44]. It should be treated by using nystatin suspension, 100 000 units/ml, 4 hourly. (Dentures should be cleaned and rinsed with nystatin also.) Nystatin pastilles, amphotericin lozenges, miconazole gel (25 mg/ml, 5–10 ml held in the mouth as long as possible, four times a day) are alternative treatments. Resistant infection may require ketoconazole, 200 mg once daily in tablets or suspension (for resistant infection a dose can be given twice a day), or fluconazole (50 mg daily, for seven to 14 days – reported to have fewer side effects than ketoconazole)[41,42] (see page 85).

Dental problems

The patient's cachexia may cause shrinkage of the gums, and dentures then become loose and irritating. Other dental problems may also need the attention of a dentist and even though life expectancy may only be a matter of a few weeks, dental care may provide much appreciated comfort for the patient. Discomfort caused by dentures or problems with teeth will affect a patient's ability to smile, talk, eat and drink and may make them embarrassed or reluctant to seek company.

Drugs

Those drugs suspected of causing mouth soreness should be withdrawn or the dosage reduced. Cytotoxic drugs frequently cause gingivitis or glossitis. Antibiotics occasionally do likewise and make a patient more susceptible to fungal infection. Tricyclic antidepressants, phenothiazines, antihistamines, and antimuscarinics (less correctly termed anticholinergics[45]) all cause dryness of the mouth, but this is usually dose-related.

Mouth dryness

This can be caused by local radiotherapy, drugs (see above), dehydration, or breathing through the mouth, and should be treated by giving the patient chopped ice, flavoured according to their taste, frequent ice-cold clear drinks, sweets to suck, cubes of fruit, pineapple to chew (a common favourite is to freeze chunks of pineapple), frequent mouth washes and artificial saliva (spray or pastilles). Foam stick applicators are useful for applying fluid and medication to the mouth and tongue.

Aphthous ulceration

Local applications of protective gel (carmellose sodium paste) or carbenoxolone gel or triamcinolone dental paste or local anaesthetic spray may help. For severe recurrent ulceration, mouthwashes of compound thymol glycerine, or tetracycline suspension mouthwash (or made by stirring the contents of a 250 mg capsule into water) held in the mouth for 2–3 minutes, three times a day for three days will help[42].

Viral infections

Herpes simplex virus is the most common, but herpes zoster, cytomegalovirus, and Epstein-Barr virus are reported. These require soft diet, adequate fluid intake and often analgesics. Acyclovir cream applied every four hours is suitable for infections of the lip but not inside the mouth or on mucous membranes. This should be applied at the first sign of infection. Tetracycline rinsed in the mouth (*see* above) may be effective. For severe infections treatment is acyclovir, orally 200 mg four times a day for herpes simplex, or 800 mg five times a day for herpes zoster, given for five to seven days[9,41,42].

Halitosis

This may be caused by poor oral hygiene but more often is due to respiratory or gastrointestinal infections or vomiting. Any underlying infection should be treated and metronidazole is used for anaerobic infections, 400 mg, three times a day. Treat also with routine mouth care and treatment for dry mouth.

Cancrum oris

The gross inflammation, ulceration and infection of cancrum oris is rarely seen nowadays. Intensive nursing care with half hourly oral toilet is needed, plus treatment of the underlying infection. Treatment for dry mouth can also be given, vitamin B complex, vitamin C, metronidazole (400 mg, three times a day) and nystatin (2 ml, 4 hourly).

Excessive salivation

Hyoscine hydrobromide given sublingually, or via a transdermal patch releasing approximately 500 μg over 72 hours, will reduce saliva.

Other Common Symptoms

Urinary problems

Retention

This can be caused by drugs, such as the antimuscarinics (anticholinergics), including hyoscine and tricyclic and related antidepressants; neurological problems, such as paraplegia; an organic obstruction, such as an enlarged prostate; tumour infiltration, or constipation.

To treat urinary retention it is usually necessary to pass a catheter, although if impacted constipation is the problem, relieving this may render catheterization unnecessary. High dose dexamethasone may be helpful if the ureter or urethra is obstructed by tumour. A stent or radiotherapy or chemotherapy may also be considered.

Urinary retention should always be considered as a possible cause of restlessness in an unconscious patient.

Frequency

Causes include infection, an enlarged prostate, bladder irritability (due to tumour, unstable bladder), diabetes, hypercalcaemia, or drugs, especially diuretics. Anxiety can also cause urinary frequency.

Specific treatments should be given as appropriate, an infection should be treated and the dose of diuretics should be reduced.

Incontinence

Patients are often acutely embarrassed and may be reluctant to mention this symptom. Causes of frequency can also lead to incontinence. Severe frequency may become incontinence if a patient is unable to get to the toilet, such as at night or because of weakness, confusion or sedation. Incontinence is also caused by fistulae (vesicovaginal or vesicorectal), neurological problems, such as an unstable or hypotonic bladder, overflow (due to urethral or catheter obstruction or any cause of urinary retention) or stress incontinence.

Treatments include:

- intensive nursing care, paying great attention to care of the skin. Emollient and barrier creams (for example, Sudocrem) can be helpful. Regular toileting and incontinence pads may be needed and privacy and dignity should be maintained at all times
- catheterization. Its purpose and procedure need to be fully explained, so that the patient can make an informed choice as to whether they wish to have a catheter or not
- intermittent self-catheterization
- desmopressin, 10–40 µg, nasally at night, for incontinence at night. For

unstable bladder, imipramine (10–20 mg, at night) or propantheline (15–30 mg, three times a day).

Diazepam and other sedative drugs are not usually given because drowsiness is likely to cause incontinence due to reduced mobility.

Some hospitals have continence advisory nurses or teams who can suggest many useful therapies and support.

Infections

These are frequent. The first sign of urinary tract infection may be apparently unrelated to the urinary tract, presenting with confusion, rigor, headache, fever, sweating, or vomiting. The urine will appear cloudy and there may be symptoms of frequency, burning and pain.

Infections usually respond to broad spectrum antibiotics, which may be given whilst awaiting the results of sensitivity investigations in the laboratory, such as trimethoprim (200 mg, twice daily) or amoxycillin (250 mg, three times a day). Short courses of antibiotics and, in some instances in women, a one day course (eg amoxycillin 3 g and repeated after 10–12 hours), will be sufficient unless the patient has recurrent infection or an abnormal genito–urinary tract. Bacteria is often found in the urine of patients with catheters but treatment is only required if the patient has symptoms.

Painful urethral spasm is helped by flavoxate (200 mg, three times daily) or oxybutynin (2.5–5 mg, twice or three times daily) or propantheline (15–30 mg, two or three times daily). All these drugs may cause dry mouth, blurred vision and may precipitate glaucoma. Flavoxate has least adverse effects but is also less effective.

Bladder wash-outs

These are not routinely necessary but are helpful should there be problems with catheter drainage caused, for example, by debris. Chlorhexidine (0.01% or 0.02%) can be used. Bladder haemorrhage may be reduced by 1% alum solutions for bladder wash-outs (*see* also Haemorrhage, page 69).

Weakness and tiredness

Local or regional weakness may be due to myopathy, cord compression, neuropathy, or intracerebral pathology, such as a cerebrovascular accident or metastases. Sudden onset weakness associated with drowsiness may be due to drugs, such as diazepam or opioids (with opioids this usually wears off after a few days), raised intracranial pressure, septicemia, hypoglycaemia, hypercalcaemia, and acute haemorrhage causing anaemia, or respiratory failure. Slower onset weakness could also be caused by the above but is more likely to be caused by cachexia, loss of sleep, hyperglycaemia (consider especially if the patient has been on corticosteroids), renal or hepatic failure, anaemia, or electrolyte abnormalities. Depression can also present with weakness[46].

If appropriate, any underlying cause should be treated. Weakness caused by extensive tumour may respond to low dose steroids, as for cachexia and anorexia[47]. Assessment by a physiotherapist, particularly if a patient has stiffness associated with weakness or arthritis, followed by a gentle scheme of physiotherapy and exercises may be helpful. Aids to daily living should be considered (see Poor mobility, below).

Poor mobility

The frustrations of diminished autonomy often produce a sense of helplessness and anger in having to be dependant on others for even minor personal requirements. This is particularly hard on those who have a proud or independent personality. Everything the patient needs or is expected to need should be placed within easy reach. Physiotherapy and occupational therapy assessment and treatment is often extremely useful in helping the patient make the most of their limited movement. (This should be considered with extreme care if a patient is at risk of a pathological fracture.) Immobile patients are at great risk of contractures, pressure sores and pneumonia, and should be assisted to change position regularly to prevent such complications and to help achieve a comfortable position. Special mattresses and other aids to prevent pressure sores (see page 60) are often essential. Gentle active or passive exercise diminishes stiffness and maintains circulation. Many aids to daily living are now available to assist patients, including walking aids and frames, light touch switches for call systems, radio and television, and bath aids. These should be provided and their use explained to both patient and family. The Disabled Living Foundation has a catalogue of useful aids and can give advice on equipment: the physiotherapist, occupational therapist, or local hospice, hospital or home care support team are also often able to help. Often these patients also want diversion and recreational activities compatible with their interests and capabilities.

Staff should be aware of the techniques of lifting immobile or weak patients, and will often require regular teaching sessions on lifting techniques and the use of hoists. Every unit should have a variety of hoists and lifting aids, so that the best method may be chosen for each patient. Staff should be aware of EC regulations and hospital guidelines.

Oedema

Generalized oedema is caused by anaemia, malnutrition, protein deficiency, renal failure, hepatic failure, cardiac failure, or drugs such as steroids. Diuretics can be helpful (eg frusemide) and are an essential treatment for pulmonary oedema.

Localized oedema may be lymphoedematous (see below) or postural –

often in a patient with weak muscles or paralysed limbs. Postural oedema can be helped by an elastic support, such as a shaped tubigrip or elastic support hose. Massage will often be of benefit, as will supporting or raising the limbs and some gentle movement[48].

Lymphoedema

This is an accumulation of lymph in the interstitial space of subcutaneous tissue. Secondary lymphoedema (ie disease not originating in the lymphatics) in terminal disease is usually caused by:

- metastatic cancer infiltrating the lymph nodes or vessels
- damage to lymph nodes or vessels from surgery or radiotherapy
- venous thrombosis
- chronic venous leg ulcers – by overloading the lymphatic system[49].

Most commonly, one or more of the limbs is affected and sometimes the adjacent quadrant of the trunk.

At the first sign of lymphoedema, any rings should be removed from all fingers and a regime of monitoring should begin. This is best done by using a special chart to record the circumference of the limb – measured at the same level and at the same time each day. A note should be made of the skin condition, looking for signs of inflammation, state of the nails, and fungus infection, especially between the toes.

Treatment for lymphoedema has improved markedly in recent years and continues to do so. The main stay of treatment includes[49, 50]:

- daily skin care – careful hygiene is essential as even small abrasions are prone to become infected. Daily washing and careful drying, particularly between the digits, should be followed by application of a moisturizing cream. Perfumed creams or lotions should be avoided as these may cause irritation
- exercise – normal use of all muscles should be encouraged as the contractions stimulate lymph flow. Slings should be avoided as far as possible, as should excessive exercise which can be harmful
- massage – this can be self-massage or by a trained nurse, physiotherapist or family member. The area to be massaged should be free from clothing, and the patient lying down. Do not apply cream or oil as these reduce contact between hand and skin. Massage, using the flat of the hand with gentle but firm strokes, should start in a normal area and move distally into the swollen area. The increase in lymphatic contractions enhances lymph flow out of infected areas into clear areas. When the front has been treated and the patient turned over, the back should be massaged in the same way. Massage of a trunk and limb takes about twenty minutes. An electric body massager can be used in the same way, on the lowest setting.

- compression bandaging – this aims to reduce the volume of the limb and improve its shape so that containment hosiery can be fitted. It is of use if the limb is awkwardly shaped or for finger swelling and if the skin is damaged or fragile where fitting hosiery may cause skin damage[49].
- containment hosiery – this will prevent fluid re-accumulating after exercise or massage. Hosiery should fit snugly and comfortably around the limb and can be worn all day but is usually removed at night
- pneumatic compression pumps – these are of limited use. They may reduce the limb volume more rapidly and help to disrupt tissue fibrosis but should not be used if there is any suspicion of venous thrombosis, if there is evidence of trunk oedema (because the fluid from the limb is simply pushed from the limb into an already congested area), or if there are extensive cutaneous metastases[49,51]. The system consists of an inflatable sleeve, connected to a motor driven air pump. The limb is inserted into the sleeve, which inflates (up to 60 mmHg) and deflates cyclically.

Drug treatment can include antibiotics, if appropriate, to treat infection. Steroids, for example, dexamethasone, 4–8 mg daily, slowly reducing the dose after a week, may facilitate lymphatic drainage by reducing tumour oedema. Anticoagulants may be necessary for venous thrombosis.

Ascites

This only needs treatment if it is causing discomfort, such as abdominal distention or dyspnoea. It is useful to monitor its progress by regular measurements of the abdominal girth. Paracentesis can give immediate relief for troublesome symptoms – such as abdominal distention pain, dyspnoea, a squashed stomach syndrome – but the fluid will recur. When draining ascites, it is better to avoid using trocar and cannula. The patient should have an empty bladder. A site is chosen in the left lower quadrant, and infiltration down to the peritoneum with 0.5% lignocaine or bupivacaine as local anaesthetic. A tiny cut is made through the skin and a small catheter (such as a suprapubic catheter, which can be connected to a drainage bag, or a peritoneal dialysis catheter) is inserted. Two litres are drained in the first hour, after which the drainage is slowed down for six to 12 hours. The catheter is then removed and a simple dressing applied. If there is seepage a colostomy bag can be placed over the site – this usually stops after one to two days.

Hypercalcaemia

This should be suspected where there are bone metastases and the patient is vomiting, nauseous, anorexic, or drowsy and confused. It has been reported in up to approximately 10% of cancer patients and is most commonly caused by cancers of the bronchus (squamous cell), breast, and myeloma, and is very rare with adenocarcinomas of the stomach and prostate.

Treatment is only necessary if there are symptoms. A first step is rehydration, which in some patients can be achieved by oral fluids; a safe alternative, especially in home care, is to infuse normal saline subcutaneously via a butterfly needle. If severe hypercalcaemia persists, biphosphonates (disodium pamidronate by slow intravenous infusion, usually giving an initial dose of 30 mg in 500 ml of normal saline over four hours, followed by doses of 16 mg in at least 125 ml of saline over two hours up to a maximum of 90 mg per single treatment) may cause calcium levels to fall after two days and to remain lower for several weeks. Oral biphosphonates, such as sodium clodronate, may occasionally be useful in preventing recurrence of hypercalcaemia and oral phosphate tablets may help if the hypercalcaemia is only mild or moderate. However, poor absorption limits their effectiveness and these tablets do cause diarrhoea. Steroids have been reported to lower calcium levels in myeloma, lymphomas, and some types of breast and renal cancers but not in solid tumours. Hormone therapy can prevent the recurrence of hypercalcaemia in hormone sensitive breast cancer[9,33].

Dehydration

Dehydration can be caused by a lack of fluid intake (due to weakness, dysphagia etc) or loss of fluid (eg from a haemorrhage or in hyperglycaemia or hypercalcaemia). Dehydration may cause thirst (especially in the early stages), dry mouth, reduced blood pressure, dark urine and lethargy. In terminal illness these often may not be a problem, and the thirst and dry mouth can be treated symptomatically (see Mouth dryness, page 61); intravenous fluids are rarely needed. Confusion caused by dehydration can be effectively treated with subcutaneous fluids (for example, subcutaneous normal saline – hypodermoclysis)[52]. In one report dehydration is thought to have an analgesic effect[53]. The lessened urinary output, reduced respiratory secretions, and reduced gastric secretions, may also enhance rather than reduce a patient's comfort[53, 54].

Haemorrhage

Patients and their families are often alarmed by any bleeding, and even small amounts of blood seeping through dressings stain clothes and bedding very quickly.

Evidence of bleeding may present as haemoptysis, haematemesis, haematuria, rectal or vaginal bleeding or bleeding from fungating lesions. Treatment by anticoagulants (such as warfarin) needs careful monitoring and should be reduced should bleeding occur. Treatment of small haemorrhages includes:

- topical application of aluminium astringents (1% alum solution, sucralfate), for fungating lesions
- capillary bleeding when changing a dressing – apply gauze soaked in

adrenaline 1:1000; calcium alginate solution reduces the likelihood of bleeding from fungating lesions
- topical tranexamic acid for rectal carcinoma
- systemic drugs, such as ethamsylate 500 mg, four times daily, or tranexamic acid (caution in haematuria, may cause hard clots/obstruction) 1 gram, three times a day
- consider radiotherapy, laser therapy, diathermy and embolization for bronchial or renal bleeding.

Bleeding in the gastrointestinal tract may be due to drugs causing gastric irritation, for example, NSAIDs. These should be treated with ulcer healing drugs, such as ranitidine.

A massive haemorrhage may be heralded by small prodromal bleeds. This also applies to haemorrhage from internal organs. Haemoptysis, haematemesis or melaena may be slight at first but may be a warning of a massive haemorrhage to come. The instinctive reaction of doctors and nurses is to do everything possible to stop the bleeding, but this is not always the appropriate treatment in terminal illness, nor are resuscitation or transfusions generally used. If a large haemorrhage is anticipated, green or red towels and drapes should be available. Sedation may be appropriate if a large haemorrhage occurs along with emotional support and care for the patient's family[55].

Excessive sweating

This may be distressing, uncomfortable and cause fluid loss. Cancers may alter normal sweating by the secretion of tumour-related humoral factors or by acting peripherally on sweat glands. Sweating is also caused by fever due to infection.

Management includes treatment of any underlying infection. If there is fever, increase skin cooling from a fan, and paracetamol or NSAIDs, such as naproxen (500 mg, twice a day). Octreotide (50 micrograms, subcutaneously twice a day) for carcinoid syndrome sweating, propranolol (40 mg, three times a day) and thioridazine have all been reported to reduce sweating in some patients. Any drugs which reduce fluid volume, for example, diuretics, should be stopped[9,32,56].

Pruritus

The threshold for this varies with the patient's mood and morale. When pruritus is severe it causes great distress and misery. Pruritus is usually worse at night or with heat or following alcohol. General management includes avoiding heat, hot baths, rough clothing; cool air helps. Common causes and management of pruritus in terminal illness are shown in Box 2.6[32,56,57].

Disfigurement

This may cause enormous mental suffering. The feeling of being repulsive is demoralizing and causes the patient to reject human contact and seek iso-

Box 2.6: Causes and management of pruritus

Possible cause	Management
Dry, flaky skin	Avoid heat, hot baths; moisturize (menthol in aqueous cream is cooling).
Wet skin, for example, incontinence	Barrier creams, keep skin dry.
Infection, cellulitis, candida, herpes	Treat infection.
Radiotherapy	Keep skin dry, hydrocortisone cream 1%.
Metastatic deposits of tumour in skin	Local radiotherapy, NSAID, consider anti-tumour therapy.
Pre-existing skin disease eg eczema, psoriasis	Treat pre-existing condition.
Irritating clothing/contact dermatitis	Cotton night-clothes, avoid irritating and rough clothing.
Jaundice	Treat as dry skin. Drug treatments which have some reports of success include: steroids, dexamethasone (2–16 mg, three times daily), stanozolol (5–10 mg daily) or mesterolone (25 mg three times daily), cholestyramine (4–8 g daily) (poorly tolerated because of unpleasant taste), and most recently, naloxone and rifampicin. Ultraviolet light may be helpful but is difficult to offer to very sick patients.
Hepatic failure	As jaundice, except cholestyramine is of no benefit.
Renal failure	As hepatic failure. Erythropoietin was effective in one trial.
Carcinoid syndrome	As dry skin, and steroids or haloperidol as for jaundice. Consider anti-tumour therapy.
Iron-deficiency anaemia	Treat anaemia, if appropriate; general measures as dry skin.
Hodgkin's and non-Hodgkin's lymphoma and melanomatosis	Treat as carcinoid syndrome. Anti-tumour therapy may help, NSAID helps. Cimetidine also reported as helpful.
Drug or food sensitivity. Allergy.	Stop food or drug responsible, if appropriate. Antihistamine.

lation. Disfigurement is particularly distressing to women and young people. It may range from a single scar, about which the patient is inordinately sensitive, to a gross fungating lesion. Cosmetics, scar covering creams and sunglasses may conceal minor blemishes. A wig may work wonders for a patient with an unsightly scalp, for example, after chemotherapy.

It is futile to attempt to conceal or ignore the gross disfigurement but it is essential to warn visitors who have not seen the condition, to be prepared and to show no sign of repugnance. Sitting close to the patient, holding hands, listening and talking, as for all patients, are helpful ways of desensitizing the patient (see also Communicating with the patient, page 3).

Smell

A foul disagreeable smell emanating from the patient is a personal embarrassment, unpleasant for relatives and visitors, for other patients and also for those caring for the patient. The usual causes are fungating lesions, infected discharges from pressure sores or fistulae, steatorrhoea, nasopharyngeal infections and halitosis.

Air fresheners may be used discreetly and deodorants can be applied to dressings. This is simple and often very effective. Infections, fungating lesions, pressure sores and halitosis should be treated as described elsewhere in this chapter. Steatorrhoea causes bulky offensive faeces and arises from deficient pancreatic secretions. It may be helped by giving Pancrex V (pancreatin, protease, lipase and amylase) two capsules with food, four times daily.

Insomnia

Rather than prescribing hypnotics routinely it is wise to enquire why the patient is not able to sleep. Insomnia is caused by a number of factors: pain, coughing, vomiting, itching, incontinence or fear of incontinence, depression, fear, and an uncomfortable environment (too hot, cold, noisy etc).

Having investigated all possible causes of insomnia and given specific treatment and reassurance as appropriate, there remain those patients who do need a hypnotic. If a patient is already accustomed to a hypnotic and it works, there is no point in changing it.

Useful drugs for night sedation are: temazepam 10 mg and 20 mg. If there is some confusion or agitation, consider chlorpromazine 25 mg or 50 mg tablet (also available as a syrup or 100 mg suppositories). See Box 2.7 for further suggestions.

Emotional and Psychiatric Problems

Psychological and emotional problems

These are common in terminal illness but are often ignored or dismissed by the patient's family and professionals. In depth discussion is often needed to identify the cause or causes of the problems and these may prove to be quite different from what one might expect. There are so many factors interwoven: these may include the family, finances, spiritual needs, guilt, anger, fear of dying or unrelieved physical symptoms. It often helps to identify and discuss the problems. The relevant chaplain or pastor and social worker can have important roles in supporting the anxious and frightened patient. A psychiatrist or psychologist will be needed for more complicated problems or to assess psychiatric morbidity such as depression or severe anxiety states.

The patient may employ a number of different defence mechanisms and coping strategies including:

- regression – becoming more child-like
- denial – to blot out or ignore some realities
- rationalization – providing an alternative everyday explanation for symptoms or feelings rather than the true one
- intellectualization – becoming theoretical (often used by doctors and nurses in painful situations)
- projection – pushing the problem on to others
- displacement – displacing emotional energy into other thoughts and activities
- introjection – looking within oneself to find solutions
- repression – unconscious suppression of painful memories
- withdrawal and avoidance – withdrawing from and avoiding painful situations.

Understanding these mechanisms can help staff to explain and empathize with a patient's behaviour (*see* The reaction and fears of the dying patient, page 14). Each individual will usually have a number of these defence mechanisms and coping strategies. These are automatic and unconscious. It is only when the mechanisms are in excess that problems occur – for example, excessive introjection can result in self-blame, isolation and depression; excessive projection can result in alienation of friends and family members or paranoid states; excessive displacement can lead to complete exhaustion followed by severe depression or anxiety[58].

The stress of prolonged illness or the shock of a recent diagnosis of terminal cancer can predispose a person to psychiatric and psychological problems, particularly if they have few external supports (for example, they live alone, have few friends, poverty), have limited communication skills (such as in learning difficulties or impaired vision or hearing), or if they have a history of mental health problems.

Fear and anxiety

Fear and anxiety in a patient are usually easy to recognize. The face generally expresses their emotions. Some patients attempt to disguise their feelings by a fixed smile which does not illuminate their eyes, and there is often a tightening of the facial muscles, particularly the forehead.

In depth discussion (see page 14) is often needed over a period of time and any causes for anxiety (such as poor pain control) should be dealt with. Some patients find comfort from living each day for what pleasures, joys and comforts can be achieved in that day, or by keeping a diary and recording their enjoyments, looking always for the positive uplifting events.

Benzodiazepines (such as diazepam, 2–5 mg, two or three times daily, or the shorter acting lorazepam) can be helpful. Benzodiazepines with a long half life, such as diazepam, are sedating and tend to accumulate in frail or elderly people, however, short-acting benzodiazepines, although less sedating, have more withdrawal phenomena. Extreme agitation may require a neuroleptic such as haloperidol, and in small doses this may also help milder anxiety. Sedating antidepressants, such as amitriptyline and dothiepin, are increasingly used in anxiety states and for anxiety accompanying depression (see below)[58]. These or imipramine are helpful if there are panic attacks[59, 60].

It is also well worth using non-drug techniques such as relaxation therapy, exercises in breathing control (especially if hyperventilation is a problem), and massage. These may allow drug treatment to be withdrawn.

Depression

Recent research suggests that, although adjustment disorders are common (25–35% of patients), a small but significant minority (5–15%) of patients become seriously depressed[59]. It often goes undetected, partly because patients do not readily volunteer the symptoms and partly because it is often difficult to decide where natural sadness ends and depression begins[61]. Too often it is assumed that depression in terminal illness is to be expected or is untreatable. Depression causes considerable suffering for the patient and their family and therefore should be rigorously treated. Depression is usually characterized by a gradual onset of the following symptoms and signs:

- depressed mood or irritability
- loss of interest and enjoyment
- agitation or retardation
- self-neglect or self-mutilation
- cognitive triad – self is worthless, outside world meaningless and future hopeless
- diurnal mood swings (low mood in the morning)
- early morning wakening
- change in behaviour – becoming indecisive, withdrawn, arguing.

Often the physical symptoms of depression such as weight loss, anorexia, fatigue and constipation cannot be used for diagnosis because these may be present due to the terminal illness. Depression should also be distinguished from an adjustment disorder – a maladaptive reaction to a stress that occurs within three months and persists for no more than three months. In this the symptoms are less specific than those of depression and often fluctuate from day to day and in general the adjustment disorder will respond to psychological support[59].

Management should include:

- consider any iatrogenic causes of depression, particularly drugs including some diuretics and antihypertensives, cimetidine, methotrexate, vinblastine, and, if possible, stop or alter these
- emotional and psychological support
- antidepressant drugs – tricyclic antidepressant drugs, starting at a low dose and gradually increasing to the therapeutic range; amitriptyline is useful if sedation is required: the newer drugs such as trazodone (sedating) and lofepramine (less sedating) are reported to have fewer antimuscarinic and cardiovascular adverse effects and so are often recommended in very elderly or debilitated patients. All antidepressants have some adverse effects, most commonly dry mouth, blurred vision, hesitancy of micturition and constipation, and it is wise to warn patients in advance of the likelihood of these symptoms. All of the antidepressants take two to three weeks to elevate mood, although patients may benefit from the anxiolytic or sedative effects much earlier. Serotonin uptake inhibitors (such as fluoxetine, 20 mg daily) also are effective antidepressants and are less sedating and have fewer antimuscarinic and cardiovascular side effects than tricyclics[58,59].

Case history

Mr J., aged 55, had been very successful at buying and selling property. Carcinoma of the larynx had been treated with surgery, radiotherapy and chemotherapy. On admission he had a nasogastric tube and a tracheostomy. He had much discomfort with infection and thrush and considerable cervical pain, all of which were relieved by a low dose of oral morphine, naproxen and a course of nystatin suspension. Fully aware of his diagnosis and prognosis, he was miserable and withdrawn. There was no family support – he was a widower with no children.

He showed no interest in recreational activities until he saw another patient making rugs. She soon taught him what to do. We then saw why he had been successful in business. Although he could not talk, he arranged to be transferred to another room, he purchased his materials more cheaply than we could, he found people to assist him and to get orders, and in no time he had a thriving rug factory in his room. He was so busy he often waved away the drug trolley.

He wrote a letter to us saying he had never been happier in his life – a remarkable statement from a successful business man, making rugs in a hospice and needing tubes to help him breathe and feed. He continued happily and contentedly for nine months, when he died peacefully in his sleep.

Not everyone would wish to spend the last few months of their lives making rugs, but it is important to study patients' interests, capabilities and wishes and do everything possible to provide whatever is appropriate.

Those who have, or have had religious convictions gain peace and tranquillity by having spiritual comfort and support from their pastors. Close co-operation between doctors, nurses and clergy can be very rewarding.

Case history

Mr F., 65 years, had advanced stage of carcinoma of the lung. Weak, but symptoms well controlled, he was up and mobile, but morose and withdrawn and fully aware of the diagnosis and prognosis. One day I said to him, 'Is there anything at all you would like us to do to help you to be more relaxed?' His reply was that he would dearly like to see his family before he died. He was a Frenchman who had come over with General de Gaulle and, after the war, married an English woman and settled in London where he had a good job. He made desultory attempts to contact his family but they had all left the family farm in the south of France and, as his interests were all in the UK, he did not persevere.

His daughter had died about five years previously. His wife had died a year ago and shortly afterwards he had developed his cancer. He now had no family in the UK, just a few friends, and he felt lonely.

He gave us the address of his old family home and we got in touch with the Hotel de Ville, the gendarmerie and the curé in the nearest town. Nobody knew of his family but they promised to make enquiries. A few days later, the gendarmerie telephoned again and gave us a contact number. We followed this up, found a brother and told him about Mr F. We arranged for two brothers to come and see Mr F. and for a charity to pay their expenses.

The following Saturday morning I witnessed their arrival. They were almost a caricature of Frenchmen – berets, moustaches, clutching bottles of wine, roars of laughter and great Gallic excitement. Mr F. was transported with joy. They stayed for three days and departed, sad, but still laughing. Mr F. died three weeks later, relaxed and peaceful.

Restoration of family contacts and reconciling family relationships are often time consuming and emotionally demanding, but are supremely worthwhile.

Confusion

A distressing symptom for patients, families and carers. There are two main types, delirium and dementia. Fear, anxiety and depression exacerbate confusion, and can occasionally present with confusion. To assist in the diagnosis of cognitive impairment, due to delirium or dementia, simple tests such as Folstein's Mini-Mental State Examination[62], or the ten item Abbreviated Mental Test Score[63] are often helpful. This test takes five minutes to test for concentration, orientation, memory and comprehension.

Delirium (acute brain syndrome)

This is potentially reversible. It can range from mild confusion to gross psychosis with hallucinations, paranoia and negativism. Its onset may be rapid but, if the cause can be identified and treated rigorously, there may be complete recovery. Its causes include toxic, eg chest and urinary tract infections (frequently delirium is the first sign of a developing infection); biochemical, eg hypercalcaemia, diabetes, uraemia, dehydration, hypoxia; drugs, eg sensitivity, excessive doses, interactions or sudden withdrawal. All medication should be reviewed and enquiries about drugs taken previously (remember alcohol) should be made. Atropine, hyoscine, diuretics, digoxin, phenytoin, benzodiazepines, and many other drugs can cause confusion. Patients who have diabetes usually require much lower doses of insulin or hypoglycaemic drugs in terminal illness, and if these drugs are continued, hypoglycaemia with acute delirium may develop rapidly.

Preferably a person familiar to the patient should be in charge of the situation and avoid crowding (a well-briefed relative may be helpful). Gentle coaxing in a calm unruffled manner often obtains co-operation. Staff should not argue or be offended by the patient's behaviour. Search for a cause and treat it effectively.

Drug treatment of confusion is shown in Box 2.7. Mild or night time confusion requires smaller doses, severe confusion and agitation will need maximum doses. If repeated doses are required medication should be given orally (PO) or subcutaneously (SC). Once the patient is stabilized the dose is then gradually reduced.

Dementia (organic brain syndrome)

This is not reversible as it is due to the destruction of neurones. Onset is insidious with progressive loss of short-term memory and personality change. Twenty per cent of those over 80 are affected to some degree. Patients are usually placid, sluggish and withdrawn, though they may be aggressive at times if something they want, or wish to do, is denied them. Progressive intellectual impairment leads to difficulty in communication, forgetting natural functions with consequent incontinence. Neurological deficiency may follow with unco-ordination and inability to feed themselves.

If a patient appears to have dementia, consider any reversible diseases which may present with cognitive impairment such as hypothyroidism, Parkinson's disease, depression, hyperglycaemia and cerebral metastases. These should be treated appropriately.

The main objective of treatment is to improve quality of life for the patient, and to support the family and carers to reduce their stress and burden. The family may find coping with the illness extremely difficult. Mental and physical stimulation should be provided for the patient and isolation avoided. Remember, however, that a person with dementia can become more confused if very many different professional carers visit them. Patients should be persuaded to do as much as possible for themselves. Staff should treat the patient with respect, and be prepared to carefully and simply explain, as often as necessary, what is happening around them. Mobility should be encouraged

Box 2.7: Drugs of value in the management of delirium[60,64,65]

Indications	Individual drugs	Dose	Special features
Agitated confusion	Haloperidol (PO, SC, IM)	Initial: 1.5–5 mg, repeated if needed. Maintenance: 0.5–5 mg 2–12 hourly	Drug of choice in treatment of delirium in those who are medically ill. Extra-pyramidal side effects may occur.
	Chlorpromazine (PO, IM) Methotrimeprazine (PO, SC)	Initial: 25–100 mg Maintenance: 12.5–50 mg, three times a day	Methotrimeprazine more sedating and may cause hypotension.
	Lorazepam (PO, IM)	0.5–2.0 mg 1–4 hourly	Combination of lorezepam and haloperidol useful for sedation. Lorezepam alone may worsen confusion.
	Midazolam (SC)	30–100 mg per 24 hours	Useful for agitation.
Paranoid confusion	Trifluoperazine	2–4 mg three times daily	Where agitation not a feature.
	Chlorpromazine	25 mg three times daily	Where agitation a feature.
Nocturnal restless/ confusion	Thioridazine	25 mg 5 pm 50 mg 9 pm (1 am dose pm)	Minimal extra-pyramidal side effects.
	Drugs above given in 5 pm and 9 pm doses also suitable help.		

and physiotherapy offered, if necessary. A good personal appearance should be maintained and regular checks on general health, especially sight, teeth, and hearing be made. Reminiscence therapy can often lift spirits and reality orientation can help to keep the mind as active as possible. For example, the environment should be as homely as possible and encourage orientation, including a calendar showing the correct date, and patients should be reminded of the place, season, and day of the week. Entertainment, individually or in groups, with music and straightforward games, with encouragement of reminiscences with family photographs and talks about their earlier lives, is often helpful.

Dementia does not respond to drug treatment, indeed, as there is a deficiency of active neurones, normal doses of psychotropic drugs may easily lead to over-sedation. Mild sedation may be required at night.

References

[1] Cartwright, A. (1991) Changes in life and care in the year before death 1969–1987. *Journal of Public Health Medicine* 13(2):81–7.

[2] Kinzbrunner, B. (1990) Letters to the editor – The role of chemotherapy in the hospice patient. *American Journal of Hospital Care*, Jan/Feb:8–11.

[3] Pagnoncelli, D., Bulcao Vianna, L. (1992) The use of chemotherapy in palliative care. *Palliative Medicine* 6:4:341–2.

[4] Higginson, I. (1993) *Clinical audit in palliative care*. Radcliffe Medical Press, Oxford.

[5] Dixon, P., Higginson, I., Chandler, S., Wade, A., McCarthy, M. (1989) Use of controlled release morphine sulphate tablets by a terminal care support team: a retrospective cohort study. *In* ed. Twycross, R. G., *The Edinburgh Symposium on Pain and Medical Education*. Royal Society of Medicine International Symposium Series (149), London, 23–34.

[6] Twycross, R. G. (1989) Cancer pain a global perspective. *In* ed. Twycross, R. G. *The Edinburgh Symposium on Pain and Medical Education*. Royal Society of Medicine International Symposium Series (149), London; 3–16.

[7] Hanks, G. and Justins, D. (1992) Cancer pain: management. *Lancet*; **339**, 1031–6.

[8] World Health Organization (1986) *Cancer pain relief*. Geneva: World Health Organization.

[9] Regnard, C., Tempest, S. (1992) *A guide to symptom relief in advanced cancer*, (3rd edition). St Oswald's Hospice, Newcastle upon Tyne.

[10] Hoskins, P. and Hanks, G. (1988) The management of symptoms in advanced cancer: experience in a hospital-based continuing care unit. *Journal of the Royal Society of Medicine*; **81**, 341–4.

[11] Sewell, G. (1992) Pharmaceutical aspects of pain control. *In* ed. Stewart, B. J. *Terminal care in the community: a guide for pharmacists*. Radcliffe Medical Press Oxford, 50–62.

[12] Kaiko, R. F., Healy, N., Pav, J., Thomas, G. B., Goldenheim, P. D. (1989) The comparative bioavailability of MS Contin tablets (controlled release morphine) following rectal and oral administration. *In* ed. Twycross, R. G., *The Edinburgh Symposium on Pain and Medical Education*. Royal Society of Medicine International Symposium Series (149), London, 235–41.

13 Thompson, J., Regnard, C. (1992) Managing pain in advanced cancer – a flow diagram. *Palliative Medicine*; 6:4:329–35.

14 Johnson, I., Patterson, S. (1992) Drugs used in combination in the syringe driver – a survey of hospice practice. *Palliative Medicine*; 6:125–30.

15 Finch, M. (1992) Intraspinal drug delivery systems. *International Cancer Nursing News*; 4:4, 4–6.

16 Ripamonti, C., Bruera, E. (1992) Transdermal and inhalatory routes of opioid administration: the potential application in cancer pain. *Palliative Medicine*; 6:98–104.

17 Portenoy, R. K. (1993) *Adjuvant analgesics in pain management. In* eds. Doyle, D., Hanks, G. W. C., MacDonald, N., *Oxford Textbook of Palliative Medicine,* 187–203; 229–44.

18 Hanks, G. W., Portenoy, R. K., MacDonald, N., O'Neill, W. M. (1993) Difficult pain problems. *In* eds. Doyle, D., Hanks, G. W. C., MacDonald, N., *Oxford Textbook of Palliative Medicine,* 257–74.

19 Thompson, J. W. and Filshie. (1993) *Transcutaneous electrical nerve stimulation (TENS) and acupuncture. In* eds. Doyle, D., Hanks, G. W. C., MacDonald, N., *Oxford Textbook of Palliative Medicine,* 229–243.

20 Higginson, I., McCarthy, M. (1989) Measuring symptoms in terminal cancer: are pain and dyspnoea controlled? *Journal of the Royal Society of Medicine*; 82: 1761–4.

21 Heyse-Moore, L., Ross, V., Mulles, M. (1991) How much of a problem is dyspnoea in advanced cancer? *Palliative Medicine*; 5:20–6.

22 Regnard, C., Ahmedzai, S. (1990) Dyspnoea in advanced cancer – a flow diagram. *Palliative Medicine*; 4(4):311–15.

23 Regnard, C., Ahmedzai, S. (1991), Dyspnoea in advanced nonmalignant disease – a flow diagram. *Palliative Medicine*; 5:56–60.

24 Heyse-Moore, L. (1993) Respiratory symptoms. *In* eds. Saunders, C. and Sykes, N. *The management of terminal malignant disease,* (3rd edition). Edward Arnold, London; 76–93.

25 Ahmedzai, S. (1993) Palliation of respiratory symptoms. *In* eds. Doyle, D., Hanks, G. W. C., MacDonald, N. *Oxford Textbook of Palliative Medicine,* 349–78.

26 Regnard, C., Comiskey, M. (1992) Nausea and vomiting in advanced cancer – a flow diagram. *Palliative Medicine*; 6:2:146–51.

27 Baines, M. and Sykes, N. (1993) Gastrointestinal symptoms. *In* eds. Saunders,

C. and Sykes, N. *The management of terminal malignant disease*, (3rd edition). Edward Arnold, London, 63–76.

[28] Sykes, N. P. (1991) A clinical comparison of laxatives in a hospice. *Palliative Medicine*; 5:307–14.

[29] Twycross, R. G. (1993) Dysphagia, dyspepsia, hiccup. *In* eds. Doyle, D., Hanks, G. W. C., MacDonald, N. *Oxford Textbook of Palliative Medicine*: 291–9.

[30] Twycross, R. G., Lack, S. A. (1986) *Control of alimenary symptoms in far advanced cancer*. Churchill Livingstone, Edinburgh.

[31] Drug and Therapeutics Bulletin (1990). Intractable hiccup: baclofen and nifedipine are worth trying. *Drug and Therapeutics Bulletin*; 28: 36.

[32] Hoy, A. Other symptom challenges. *In* eds. Saunders, C. and Sykes, N. *The management of terminal malignant disease*, (3rd edition). Edward Arnold, London: 160–8.

[33] Dunlop, R. (1993) Metabolic symptoms. *In* eds. Saunders, C. and Sykes, N., *The management of terminal malignant disease*, (3rd edition). Edward Arnold, London, 94–101.

[34] Brennan M. F., Total parenteral nutrition in the cancer patient, *New England Journal of Medicine*, 305:373–5.

[35] DeWys, W. D., Begg, D., Lavin, P. T. (1980) Prognosis effect of weight loss prior to chemotherapy in cancer patients. *American Journal of Medicine*; 69: 491–9.

[36] Tisdale, M. J. (1991) Cancer cachexia. *British Journal of Cancer*; 63:337–42.

[37] Shaw, C. (1992) Nutritional aspects of advanced cancer. *Palliative Medicine*; 6: 105–10.

[38] Bruera, E., MacDonald, R. N. (1988) Nutrition in cancer patients: an update and review of our experience. *Journal of Pain and Symptom Management*; 3: 133–40.

[39] Bruera, E., Fainsinger R. L., (1993) Clinical Management of cachexia and anorexia. *In* eds. Doyle, D., Hanks, G. W. C., MacDonald, N., *Oxford Textbook of Palliative Medicine*; 330–337.

[40] Goldstone, L. A. and Goldstone, J. (1982) The Norton Score: an early warning of pressure sores. *Journal of Advanced Nursing*; 7: 419–26.

[41] Lethem, W. (1993) Mouth and skin problems. *In* eds. Saunders, C. and Sykes, N. *The management of terminal malignant disease*, (3rd edition). Edward Arnold, London, 139–48.

[42] Ventafridda, V., Ripamonti, C., Sbanotto, A., De Conno, F. (1993) Mouth-care. In eds. Doyle, D., Hanks, G. W. C., MacDonald, N., *Oxford Textbook of Palliative Medicine*: 434–47.

[43] Finlay, I. G. (1986) Oral symptoms and candida in the terminally ill. *British Medical Journal*; **293**: 592–3.

[44] De Gregorio, M. W. *et al.* (1984) Fungal infections in patients with acute leu-kaemia. *American Journal of Medicine*; **73**:543–8.

[45] British Medical Association and Royal Pharmaceutical Society of Great Bri-tain (1993), *British National Formulary* (Number 25). British Medical Associ-ation and Royal Pharmaceutical Society of Great Britain, London.

[46] Regnard, C., Mannix, K. (1992) Weakness and fatigue in advanced cancer – a flow diagram. *Palliative Medicine*; **6**:253–6.

[47] Bruera, E., MacMillan, K., Hanson, J., Kuehn, N., MacDonald, R. N. (1990) A controlled trial of megestrol acetate pm appetite, caloric intake, nutritional status and other symptoms in patients with advanced cancer. *Cancer*; **66**: 1279–82.

[48] O'Gorman, B. (1993) Physiotherapy in Palliative Medicine. In eds. Saunders, C. and Sykes, N. *The management of terminal malignant disease*, (3rd edi-tion). Edward Arnold, London: 168–73.

[49] Badger, C., Twycross, R. (1988) *Management of Lymphoedema*. Sir Michael Sobell House, Churchill Hospital, Oxford.

[50] Regnard, C., Badger, C., Mortimer, P. (1988) Lymphoedema – advice on treat-ment, *BLIG*, Beaconsfield.

[51] Mortimer P. S., Badger, C., Hall, J. G., (1993) Lymphoedema. In eds. Doyle, D., Hanks, G. W. C., MacDonald, N. *Oxford Textbook of Palliative Med-icine*, 407–415.

[52] Bruera, E., Legris, M. A., Kuehn, N., Miller, M. J. (1990) Hypodermoclysis for the administration of fluids and narcotic analgesics in patients with advanced cancer. *Journal of Pain and Symptom Management*; 5:218–20.

[53] Printz, L. (1989) Withholding hydration in the terminally ill: is it valid? *Geria-tric Medicine*; **19**(4):81–4.

[54] Antonowich, R. A. (1989) Dehydration and the terminally ill. *American Jour-nal of Palliative Care*; Sep/Oct:48.

[55] Regnard, C., Makin, W. (1992) Management of bleeding in advanced cancer – a flow diagram. *Palliative Medicine*; **6**:1:74–8.

[56] Hull, F. (1990) Palliative care: physical symptoms II. *Journal of Clinical Pharmacology and Therapeutics*, 15: 463–7.

[57] Bain, V. G., Minuk G. Y. (1993) Jaundice, ascites and hepatic encephalopathy. *In* eds. Doyle, D., Hanks, G. W. C., MacDonald, N. *Oxford Textbook of Palliative Medicine*, 337–348.

[58] Hodgson, G. (1993). Depression, sadness and anxiety. *In* eds. Saunders, C. and Sykes, N. *The management of terminal malignant disease*, (3rd edition). Edward Arnold, London: 102–30.

[59] Cody, M. (1990) Depression and the use of antidepressants in patients with cancer. *Palliative Medicine*; 4:4:271–8.

[60] Breitbart, W. and Passik, S. D. (1993) Psychiatric aspects of palliative care. *In* eds. Doyle, D., Hanks, G. W. C., MacDonald, N. *Oxford Textbook of Palliative Medicine*, 609–627.

[61] Maguire, P. (1980) Monitoring the quality of life in cancer patients and their relatives. *In* Symington, T., Williams, A. E., McVie, J. G. (Eds.). *Cancer: assessment and monitoring*. Churchill Livingstone, London: 40–52.

[62] Folstein, S. E., McHugh, P. R. (1975) Mini-mental state: a practical method for grading the cognitive state of patients for the clinician. *Journal of Psychiatric Research*; 53:2250–5.

[63] Power, D., Kelly, S., Gilsenan, J. *et al*. (1993) Suitable screening tests for cognitive impairment and depression in the terminally ill – a prospective prevalence study. *Palliative Medicine*; 7: 213–8.

[64] West, T. (1992) Palliative care. *In* ed. Stewart, B. J. *Terminal Care in the community: a guide for pharmacists*. Radcliffe Medical Press, Oxford: 21–49.

[65] Back, I. N. (1992) Terminal restlessness in patients with malignant diseases. *Palliative Medicine*; 6: 293–8.

Further reading

Farr, W. (1990) The use of corticosteroids for symptom management in terminally ill patients. *American Journal of Hospital Care*; Jan/Feb:41–6.

Hanks, G. W., Trueman, T., Twycross, R. G. (1983) Corticosteroids in terminal cancer – a prospective analysis of current practice. *Postgraduate Medicine*; 59:702–706.

Needham, P., Daley, A., Lennard, R. (1992) Steroids in advanced cancer: a survey of current practice. *British Medical Journal*; 305:999.

See also Further Reading, page 99.

3 | Care for Patients with Advanced AIDS and HIV Disease

Introduction

People who are infected with the human immunodeficiency virus (HIV) undergo a slow progressive suppression of immune function. Within the first few weeks following infection there will usually be a short influenza like illness with fever and, sometimes, a rash during which sero-conversion takes place. Following this there is a variable period of months or years (as long as 10–15 in a small number of cases) during which the person remains well, but is capable of transmitting infection, sexually or through blood. During this period the person will be classified as being asymptomatic HIV antibody positive.

The virus load then begins to increase, probably as the result of one or more 'trigger factors' which stimulate viral replication, and which results in a progressive destruction of the T-helper cells carrying the CD4 molecule. Measurements of immune function are usually expressed as the CD4 count; other factors such as CD4:CD8 ratio, $ß_2$ microglobulin levels, and neopterin levels are also used as markers for progression to symptomatic HIV disease or AIDS.

As the CD4 levels fall and the immune suppression progresses, the person begins to develop non-specific problems, such as weight loss, diarrhoea, persistent generalized lymphodenopathy and fevers or oral thrush. AIDS is diagnosed with the development of certain opportunistic infections, cancers such as Kaposi's sarcoma, specific HIV related problems such as HIV-encephalopathy (or AIDS-related dementia) or the HIV wasting syndrome. Advanced HIV disease, without the development of specific conditions which give an AIDS diagnosis, may also cause considerable debility, illness and indeed death.

Palliative care in patients with advanced AIDS or HIV disease include the following special features:

- the sudden changes which sometimes occur in a patient's condition
- the number of co-existing diagnoses, all causing their own problems, and usually requiring treatment, maintenance or prophylactic therapies
- polypharmacy as a result of the above
- the need for very active palliation or maintenance treatment with, for ex-

ample, IV infusions for some opportunistic infections which may cause pain or distressing symptoms

- the changing pattern of the disease and of treatment
- the youth of the majority of patients
- the isolation, stigma and lack of compassion that so many patients, and their carers, experience
- the complex social problems so many have, including homelessness and lack of family or other support structures
- the awareness that so many patients have of the disease, the current research and the funding available.

Common Opportunistic Infections

Oral and oesophageal candida

Oral candida is very common, and is an indicator of the progress from asymptomatic to symptomatic HIV disease. Oesophageal candida is an AIDS indicator disease and may be difficult to control in end-stage disease. It is characterized by anorexia, dysphagia, retrosternal discomfort or pain, and nausea or vomiting. Oral candida is usually treated with fluconazole (the drug of choice) 150 mg daily (or ketoconazole or itraconazole). Once under control, prophylaxis is usually with 50 mg daily, or 1–3 times per week. Oesophageal candida usually requires higher dosages, such as 200 mg bd, together with symptom-control. If there is severe retrosternal pain, ulceration caused by cytomegalovirus or herpes simplex infection or by a lymphoma, should be excluded.

Cytomegalovirus infection (CMV)

CMV commonly causes retinitis which may progress to blindness if untreated or, in some cases, in spite of treatment with ganciclovir or foscarnet. The appearance of the retina is typical and said to resemble a 'cheese and tomato pizza' when haemorrhages have occurred. Diagnosis should be confirmed by an experienced ophthalmologist as less acute presentations may be confusing. Any visual problems should be taken seriously and dealt with promptly. The usual treatment is by ganciclovir or foscarnet IV daily for two to three weeks, followed by maintenance treatment by IV infusion 3–5 times weekly. These infusions are maintained even in end-stage disease, or in the terminal situation, as fear of blindness, or increasing visual deficit clearly detracts from whatever quality of life is possible.

CMV may also cause colitis with abdominal pain and distension, sometimes with fresh bleeding from the intestinal mucosa, perhaps as a result of ulceration. CMV sometimes causes oesophageal ulceration with severe retrosternal pain and dysphagia. Both of these conditions are treated with IV ganciclovir or foscarnet, but the patient does not usually remain on maintenance therapy, as with retinitis. Disseminated CMV infection and CMV pneumonitis may also occur in end-stage disease.

Mycobacterial disease

Mycobacterium tuberculosis associated with HIV infection is emerging as a major health problem in many developing countries where tuberculosis already kills three million people annually. HIV may trigger a latent tuberculosis. In the West, pulmonary tuberculosis is more common in drug users with HIV than in other infected patients. Atypical forms of mycobacterial disease, such as Mycobacterium avium complex (intracellulare) causing disseminated disease, are not uncommon in advanced HIV disease. There has been an increasing incidence of multi-drug resistance in the USA since 1990, and this is also being found in other areas of the world.

Patients with mycobacterial disease may have sputum negative smears and reduced skin reactions to Mantoux testing, so diagnosis may be difficult. Symptoms include cough, weight loss, diarrhoea, anaemia, fever and severe sweats. Patients are sometimes treated empirically in order to control the above symptoms or started on antituberculous prophylaxis with isoniazid; treatment is usually with three or four antituberculous drugs such as rifabutin, ethambutol, pyrazinamide or clarithromycin. Side effects include nausea, skin rashes and abdominal pain; some patients may benefit from a short break from medication if nausea is difficult to control. Haloperidol may be more effective than other antiemetics in controlling drug-induced nausea.

The patient becomes increasingly tired, anorexic and weak, with recurrent anaemia as the degree of immuno suppression increases with the dissemination of the mycobacterium through blood and bone marrow. A blood transfusion may be effective for some weeks initially, but at the end-stage will make little difference to the patient's quality of life. Symptomatic treatment then becomes more important with supportive care.

Toxoplasmosis

Ingested cysts of toxoplasma gondi are released in the gastro intestinal tract and in the tachyzoite form, spread through the blood stream to all tissues. Abscesses are formed and the commonest presentation is with signs of one or more intracerebral lesions causing focal neurological signs. Definitive diagnosis is by brain biopsy, but a CT or MRI scan is usually sufficient to indicate the need for treatment. Differential diagnosis includes cerebral lymphoma or progressive multifocal leucoencephalopathy. A trial of treatment for three weeks is followed by a further scan; if there is a change the treatment will be continued for a further three weeks, followed by maintenance treatment for life. Treatment is commonly with pyrimethamine and sulphadiazine with folic acid or with clindamycin, or more recently, with atovaquone. In end-stage disease, the infection may be reactivated in spite of continuing prophylaxis. Headaches, nausea, vomiting and focal neurological signs may then require symptom control along usual lines. Dexamethasone may improve the headache and symptoms, but will of course mask the progress of the disease for a while.

Pneumocystis carinii pneumonia (PCP)

PCP can only be diagnosed definitively by identification of the organism on microscopy in sputum usually through bronchoscopy or broncho-alveolar lavage or induced sputum. It is the presenting illness in many patients, and may recur several times during the progress of the disease. The first episode is no longer associated with a high mortality and patients are often on primary or secondary prophylaxis with co-trimoxazole daily, or several times a week, or pentamidine by nebulizer every two to four weeks. Dapsone is also effective as a prophylaxis.

In end-stage disease invasive diagnostic tests may be inappropriate. There is usually a fever with a dry, unproductive cough and increasing dyspnoea but few chest signs. Symptom control measures should include control of cough and anxiety, and relief of the dyspnoea, all of which may be best dealt with by morphine orally, or via the syringe driver.

Diarrhoea

Diarrhoea is common throughout the course of the disease, and may be an early sign of developing symptomatic HIV disease. Causes of diarrhoea are shown in Box 3.1.

Box 3.1: Causes of diarrhoea

● Protozoa	– Cryptosporidium
	– Giardia lamblia
	– Entamoeba histolytica
	– Isospora belli
● Bacteria	– Salmonella
	– Shigella
	– Campylobacter
● Viruses	– CMV
	– Herpes simplex
	– HIV
● Mycobacteria	– MAI
	– M.Tb.

Microsporidia have recently been identified as a cause for persistent diarrhoeas; KS (intestinal) and lymphomas may also cause diarrhoea.

Whenever possible, the cause of the problem should be treated. However, recurrence is common, and eradication of the organism, eg cryptosporidium, may be very difficult. In cryptosporidiosis there is also extensive destruction of the mucosal villi in the small intestine, resulting in continuing large volume watery diarrhoea, even when the organism has been eliminated.

Continuing symptomatic treatment is often necessary as persistent diarrhoea leads to weight loss, anxiety about going out and to general misery. Loperamide is the drug of choice as it may be given in larger doses than normally recommended, up to a maximum of 32 mg/24 hours in divided doses, without any central nervous system side effects. It should be given 2–4 times daily. Sometimes the addition of a bulking agent (to reduce the wateriness of the stool) eg an ispaghula husk preparation (Fybogel) or kaolin is helpful, as may be the addition of an antispasmodic, such as Buscopan (hyoscine butylbromide). If these measures are ineffective consider using an opiate such as morphine sulphate, either as elixir, or as tablets, or in its sustained release form, but it may be that intestinal transit time is such that absorption is not taking place. In this case oral medication will be ineffective and diamorphine via a syringe driver together with an antiemetic will be necessary to obtain control. Once reasonable control has been achieved it may be possible to revert to oral medication. Vomiting may also be a problem with cryptosporidial diarrhoea and a similar approach may be necessary.

Herpes simplex

Herpes simplex infections are common and cause oral, oesophageal or anorectal and vaginal ulceration which may be very painful. Anorectal infection may cause severe pain on defaecation with tenesmus. Treatment of the infection should be started immediately with acyclovir 400 mg x 5 daily for 5–10 days, but application of local acyclovir cream may also speed resolution. Local anaesthetic gel and analgesia is also helpful and the tenesmus may be eased with chlorpromazine 25 mg tds, or with nifedipine 10 mg capsule taken at the time. The patient should bite the capsule, releasing the liquid contents to be absorbed directly through the oral mucosa, giving quick relief. Oesophageal HS ulceration may cause dysphagia and retrosternal burning and pain. Again, the treatment of the cause is the most effective measure in dealing with the symptoms, but antacids such as Mucaine or Gaviscon may ease discomfort.

Herpes zoster

Herpes zoster infections, causing chickenpox or shingles, is common and may also cause post-herpetic neuralgia which is usually well controlled with carbamazepine. Shingles may recur and affect more than one dermatome.

Cryptococcal meningitis

The yeast cryptococcus neoformans causes a severe meningitis which may present acutely, but which recurs or becomes chronic following initial treatment. The treatment of choice, which is very effective, is now fluconazole given in high doses intravenously followed by oral maintenance therapy with 400 mg daily or bd. Persistent or recurring headaches are a common feature and may be difficult to treat. Codeine phosphate, 60 mg, 6 hourly, may be effective, but will have its own side-effects such as constipation.

Skin infections

These are very common (*see* table 3.1).

HIV-Related Neurological problems

These are extremely common, at postmortem having been identified in about 90% or more cases. The causes range from opportunistic infections such as toxoplasmosis, cryptococcal, mycobacterial and viral infections to cerebral lymphoma and HIV itself.

Progressive multi-focal leuko-encephalopathy (PML)

PML occurs in a small percentage of patients and is caused by the JC virus of the papova group. Multiple lesions in the white matter cause focal or diffuse signs, and the disease usually progresses quickly. There is no effective treatment, but symptomatic therapy and supportive care are, of course, very important for the patient as well as for the family and partner as the deterioration progresses.

HIV encephalopathy or AIDS dementia complex (ADC)

This is directly attributable to HIV. AZT (Zidovudine) has been shown to delay its onset, and even to improve it in the early stages for some time.

Differential diagnosis may be very difficult in the early stages. A CT or MRI scan may show no cerebral atrophy, or very little, even when other signs are fairly clear. Psychometric testing may be helpful, and other treatable causes of confusion or memory loss must be excluded. Bizarre behaviour and personality changes may require psychiatric input, and sensitive, supportive care for the patient, partner and family are needed to help them cope with the anxiety and distress that is inevitable. The patient may become very anxious because the intermittent nature of the confusion often means that he is aware that he is confused. Patients with HIV encephalopathy appear to become particularly sensitive to psychotropic drugs, and these should be used cautiously to start with.

Table 3.1: Common skin problems[1]

Condition	Cause	Treatment
Dry skin	Malnutrition due to persistent diarrhoea causing reduced triglycerides	Control of diarrhoea, and nausea and vomiting; diet and appetite stimulants; emollients
Seborrhoeic dermatitis	Often associated with fungal or yeast infections	Topical steroids and antifungal creams, Selsun shampoo, Betnovate scalp lotion
Folliculitis (generalized pruritic eruption)	Often associated with fungal or yeast infections	Antihistamines, Eurax (Crotamiton) NB exclude scabies
Psoriasis	May appear for first time in HIV + ve person	Salicyclic acid, coal tar, dithranol and strong topical steroids
Molluscum contagiosum	Pox virus	Phenol or silver nitrate applications, cryotherapy
Ringworm	Tinea	Fluconazole, itraconazole, griseofulvin and antifungal creams
Norwegian scabies or crusted scabies	Very high number of scabies mites in immuno-compromised individual; delay in diagnosis	Gamma benzene hexachloride applications x 3 initially followed by weekly applications for several months; possible need for strong topical steroids to reduce skin reactions

Table 3.2: HIV encephalopathy[1]

Early signs	Short-term memory loss intermittent confusion loss of concentration changes in personality and behaviour
Progress of encephalopathy	Diffuse neurological signs ataxia tremor limb weaknesses loss of co-ordination
Advanced encephalopathy	Total dementia Incontinence Grand mal attacks

Peripheral neuropathy

Peripheral neuropathy is thought to be due to HIV, and often presents with tingling (or pins and needles), numbness or shooting pains in the toes, soles of feet and up the legs. It may cause marked loss of mobility due to the discomfort or pain on walking, and some patients will have to use a wheelchair if it is not controlled. Good control is usually possible with carbamazepine, starting at 100 mg bd, or with sodium valproate.

When the main sensation is one of burning, then amitriptyline 25 mg bd or tds may be effective; in some instances the anticonvulsant combined with the tricyclic antidepressant will be more effective. In difficult cases, the addition of a non-steroidal anti-inflammatory or of an opiate such as morphine sulphate may improve the pain-control; and the topical application of a capsaicin containing cream may also be effective.

HIV-Related Cancers

Kaposi's sarcoma (KS)

KS is the most common cancer in AIDS and occurs more commonly in sexually transmitted HIV infection. There may be an additional transmissible factor involved but this has not been proven. AIDS-related KS presents with isolated raised reddish-purple cutaneous lesions which do not usually cause pain, but may be distressing due to their visibility, especially on the face. Camouflage make-up (advice through the Red Cross) may help for a time. Radiotherapy will effectively deal with isolated lesions on the face or elsewhere in the earlier stages. As the disease progresses, and the number of KS lesions increases, other problems develop with local pain and ulceration or lymphoedema; weight loss and fever (with no other cause) may also become evident. KS may also develop viscerally, in the gastrointestinal mucosa including the oesophagus and in the palate and gums, and in the lungs. Chemotherapy may be very effective in controlling or reducing the KS up to a point. Patients who do not succumb to other causes of AIDS-related death, will eventually develop very extensive disseminated KS. Ulceration, sometimes following radiotherapy, may cause severe pain, and good wound management together with analgesia is essential. A non-steroidal anti-inflammatory drug with appropriate opiate therapy will usually give good control, and orofacial oedema may respond dramatically to dexamethasone.

The patient will be very distressed by his or her appearance, and will sometimes be very self-conscious and feel great self-disgust. It is essential for the carer not to compound this by showing reluctance to approach or touch the patient. Much sensitive support will be needed. In end-stage disease, with widely disseminated KS, the skin may break down easily, and the patient should be nursed on an appropriate mattress to prevent the development of pressure areas.

Lymphomas

The commonest type which occurs in AIDS is the high grade ß-cell lymphoma. The most common sites are in the CNS, bone marrow, gastrointestinal tract, liver, heart, lungs and lymph nodes. Good rates of temporary remission are being achieved with chemotherapy, but the overall prognosis remains poor.

Primary cerebral lymphomas

Primary cerebral lymphomas are the cause of death in an increasing though still small number of patients with AIDS as median survival times are lengthening with improved treatments. Differential diagnosis include toxoplasmosis and PML, but presentation is usually with focal neurological signs. Definitive diagnosis is by brain-biopsy, but as prognosis is poor in any case, even with radiotherapy, this is often not performed. If toxoplasmosis is suspected, a trial of treatment is usually attempted for 2–3 weeks, with a follow-up scan to monitor response. Radiotherapy may give an initial response, but symptomatic treatment for headaches, nausea, vomiting, and control of seizures are essential for maintenance of quality of life for as long as possible.

Pain in AIDS

More than 60% of patients with advanced HIV or AIDS develop severely painful conditions. The causes include KS, lymphomas, opportunistic infections and HIV itself. Peripheral neuropathy is the most common painful condition associated directly with HIV. Herpes simplex and CMV ulceration can both cause severe pain, as may intracranial conditions such as a lymphoma or meningitis. It is important whenever possible, to identify and to treat the cause as part of pain management. The basic principles of pain control in cancer should be applied to the control of pain in AIDS. The same principles apply to dealing with other symptoms common in anyone with a terminal illness.

Death Certificates and Body Bags

The stigma, prejudice and fear which still surround this disease have resulted in the development by many doctors and hospital personnel of a high standard of confidentiality, and of special ways of protecting the patients and their families from the public. One of these involves the death certificate. In Britain this is a public document, open to any newspaper journalist or other interested party. Until the public attitude to HIV and AIDS changes many doctors will continue to avoid writing AIDS on a death certificate if the patient or the next of kin wish it. In order to ensure true statistical information reaching the appropriate bodies a separate letter may be sent in confidence. Alternatively, a box on the back of the death certificate inviting further enquiry may be ticked.

The Department of Health guidelines state that the body of someone with HIV infection must be placed after death in a plastic body bag with 'Risk of infection' labels attached, both to the body and to the bag.

It is important that the health care professionals concerned with the particular patient or family have some idea as to the attitudes of local funeral directors to dealing with such bodies. Unnecessary distress has been caused to families and partners when funeral directors have refused to be involved at the last minute on finding out about the diagnosis.

References

[1] Sims R. and Moss V., (1991) *Terminal care for people with AIDS*. Edward Arnold, London.
See also Further Reading, page 99.

4 | Physiology of Dying

To describe the process of dying an appropriate starting point is the time when active efforts to cure the patient's illness have ceased and the doctor has decided as a result of clinical examination that the advent of death is not far away and that continuing care of the patient is concerned entirely with relieving distressing symptoms and ensuring that the remaining few days, weeks or months of the patient's life are comfortable.

The five vital systems of the body – the cardiovascular, pulmonary, gastrointestinal, renal and central nervous systems have complex, mutually supporting interactions and if one system breaks down there is a knock-on effect on the other systems. As the deficiencies multiply a constantly changing kaleidoscope of symptoms develops. We know we cannot cure the patient and our concern is therefore to ensure by palliative care that none of these symptoms causes distress.

Causes of Death

Once a patient has entered the terminal phase it must be accepted that sudden death is always a possibility and the relatives should be forewarned accordingly and at the same time given a full but simplified explanation of the patient's illness.

There may be a sudden internal or external haemorrhage due to tumour, erosion of a major blood vessel, a massive embolus affecting the lungs or brain, severe heart failure or acute pulmonary oedema.

It is more usual for the patient to move gradually towards the closing stages of life by progressive dysfunction of one or more of the major systems.

The Cardiovascular System

Abnormalities within the heart itself, eg coronary disease may cause arrhythmias. There may be diminution of circulatory volume as in shock or haemorrhage. A breakdown of the other systems will also affect heart action, eg electrolytic disturbances or severe anaemia. The resultant defective pumping action of the heart in turn leads to hypoxia elsewhere.

Major resuscitative procedures are irrelevant for the heart failure supervening in terminal illness. It suffices to concentrate on controlling whatever symptoms arise which are distressing to the patient.

The Pulmonary System

Defective oxygenation from pulmonary dysfunction may arise from: infection; tumour infiltration; bronchospasm or asthma; oedema; effusion; pneumothorax or infarct.

Specific symptomatic treatment should provide considerable relief from any distress occasioned by these conditions, but there remains a probability of the development of cerebral hypoxia. A common cause of death is infection leading to pneumonia.

The Gastrointestinal and Renal Systems

Obstructions, infections, tumour infiltration and liver or renal failure may cause various toxic and electrolytic disturbances affecting heart and brain function. Uraemia, in particular, is common.

The Central Nervous System

It is on the activity of the nervous system that the integrity of the personality of the individual depends. The brain and spinal cord (being enclosed in a rigid bony structure) are particularly vulnerable to any condition causing increased pressure or occupying extra space. The factors that can damage the central nervous system are: infections, eg meningitis, encephalitis, brain abscess; blood vessel disruption or obstruction, eg thrombosis, haemorrhage, emboli; toxic and metabolic disorders, eg from renal or liver failure or extraneous poisons such as drugs; malignant tumours – primary or metastatic, and hypoxia due to circulatory or pulmonary failure. Hypoxia and defective blood circulation in the brain lead to the accumulation of toxic metabolites such as lactic acid. This is a major cause of brain death as this process initiates swelling which raises intracranial pressure and further reduces the circulation and oxygen supply.

The signs of central nervous system dysfunction are, in progression: confusion and disorientation; lethargy and apathy; stupor; semi-coma and coma.

The deterioration is usually uneven and there are often marked fluctuations from one state to another.

Postural effects correlating with the brain damage may take the form of various types of paralysis, eg hemiparesis or spasticity of a limb or limbs.

Decorticate posture occurs in lethargy and stupor. Stimulation of the patient causes lower limb extension with toe pointing and upper limb flexion.

Decerebrate posture is associated with deeper unconsciousness – legs and arms extended and the palms are turned outwards.

In semi-coma the electroencephalogram changes in response to sensory stimulation. In what is called deep coma, there is no response to sensory stimuli but cortical rhythms persist in a relatively stable pattern. In terminal coma which is often seen in the final hour before respiration ceases, the cortical rhythm gradually melts into an isoelectric state which, however, is still not necessarily irreversible.

As brain hypoxia worsens the pupils dilate and eventually become unresponsive to light. The blood pressure falls and the pulse becomes rapid, feeble and irregular. Occasionally convulsive seizures may occur. Cheyne-Stokes breathing is very common with cerebral hypoxia and the rapid breathing is interrupted by periods of apnoea which becomes more and more prolonged.

Approaching Death

No patient at this stage should ever be left alone. Someone sitting quietly holding the patient's hand will give great comfort and support. This is a time when family or friends are usually in constant watchful attendance. They should be kept fully informed about what is happening; for instance changing patterns of breathing and the nature and purpose of any treatment being given. The anguish of their grief will need constant support throughout this period, especially in the immediate aftermath of death.

Restlessness at this stage may be due to withdrawal reactions of the patient's medication when opioids have been suddenly discontinued. If the patient cannot take the medication orally it should be given by injection although a slightly reduced dose may suffice.

Faecal impaction should not have been allowed to develop but it may be a cause of much discomfort (see under Constipation). Urinary retention is a common cause of restlessness and may be easily overlooked – catheterization will be necessary. Lying in an awkward position or on a pressure sore will obviously cause discomfort. Extreme dryness of the mouth and/or eyes is also uncomfortable. Moisturizing with methylcellulose applications is very soothing.

Noisy breathing (the death rattle) is due to secretions in the trachea and larynx which the patient is unable to cough up. If copious, suction will help and the patient should be placed well onto one side so that the secretions can drain away. A subcutaneous injection of hyoscine 0.4 mg may also be helpful or if there is pulmonary oedema, frusemide may be necessary. If restlessness continues useful agents are listed in Box 2.7.

Signs of Death

These are absence of pulse and respiration and confirmed by absence of auscultatory sounds over the heart and trachea for at least five minutes. The pupils are fixed and dilated, and the fundi oculi show fragmentation of blood in the retinal veins.

Criteria for Diagnosis of Brain-Stem Death

Total loss of brain-stem function occurs when there are no spontaneous movements; no abnormal postures, ie no decorticate posturing, no decerebrate posturing; no epileptic jerking (these movements arise in the cortex and are routed through the brain-stem); no spontaneous respiration; no brain-stem reflexes ie no pupillary response to light, absent corneal reflex and no vestibula-ocular reflexes. Any deviation of the eyes (or even of one eye) in response to irrigation of the tympanic membrane with ice-cold water implies live cells in the brain-stem; no facial movement in response to trigeminal input (firm supraorbital pressure); no oculo-cephalic reflexes (the presence of 'doll's head' eye movement implies live cells in the brain-stem); no gag reflex.

All brain-stem reflexes must be absent before brain-stem death can be diagnosed.

Rigor mortis is a contraction of muscle, so firm as to immobilize the joints, generally appearing in two to four hours after death, attaining its full intensity within 48 hours. It begins in the jaw spreading downwards to involve the whole body and it disappears in the reverse direction. The time development is shortened in a warm atmosphere and when death occurs at a time of marked muscular activity. Reduction in adenosine triphosphate (ATP) is the chemical event that precipitates rigor mortis.

Transplants

Patients occasionally express a wish to donate their bodies for medical research. They should be asked to put this in writing, or if that is impossible, to make their wishes known verbally before two witnesses, and this should then be documented in the case notes.

HM Inspector of Anatomy[1] should be contacted. Pathological details will be required and if these prove acceptable instructions will be given as to the procedure when the patient dies.

Major transplants are usually obtained from young healthy people who have died from trauma.

Kidneys for transplant are much sought after. Contact the nearest renal unit before the patient dies if the patient has agreed or has signed a donor card.

Organs are not accepted from patients who have disseminated malignant disease.

Corneal transplants are very useful but they are only taken from patients free from eye disease and under 70 years of age. The eyes need to be removed within 36 hours. Ideally the local eye hospital should be alerted before the patient dies. Corneal transplants are acceptable in patients with malignant disease provided that the eyes have not been involved in the disease process.

Further reading

Metther, F. A. (1980) *Life and Death*. Bull, N. Y. acad med Vol 56 no. 6 p513–537.
Shakespeare, *Henry VII* 3 Death of Falstaff.

Hippocrates – Prognostics, Aphorisms.

See also Further Reading, page 99.

[1] H. M. Inspector of Anatomy Department of Health 158–176 Great Portland Street London W1N 5TB.

Further Reading

British Medical Association (1992) Statement on advance directives. BMA, London.

Cassidy, Sheila, (1988) *Sharing the darkness – the spirituality of caring*. Darton, Longman and Todd, London.

Eisenhower, J. (1982) *Poetry within hospice*. St Joseph's Hospice, London.

Ellis, B. (1981) *The long road back*. Mayhew – The Crimmon.

Frampton, D. (1986) Art in hospices. *British Medical Journal*. 293:1593–5.

Griffin, J. (1991) *Dying with dignity*. Office of Health Economics, London.

Hanratty, J. F. (1992) *Implications of legalized euthanasia*. St Joseph's Hospice, London.

Jones, R. V. H., *et al.* (1993) Death from Cancer at Home: the carer's perspective. *British Medical Journal*. 306: 249–51.

Kubler-Ross, E. (1970) *On death and dying*. Tavistock Publications, London.

O'Connor, Father Tom, *Pastoral care for the dying*. St Joseph's Hospice, London.

Parkes, C. M. (1985) Terminal care: home, hospital or hospice? *Lancet*. 155–7.

Parkes, C. M. (1986) *Bereavement: studies of grief in adult life*. Penguin, London.

Penson, Jenny, (1990) *Bereavement – a guide for nurses*. Harper and Row, London.

Pincus, Lily, (1975) *Death in the family: the importance of mourning*. Faber and Faber, London.

Report of Health Services Working Group (1990) *Hospice care in definitions and qualifications*. Help the Hospices, London.

Robbins, J., (ed.) (1989) *Care for the dying patient in the family*. Harper and Row, London.

Saunders, C. (1992) *Catholic Medical Quarterly.* 3:9–13.

Saunders, C. (1984) *Management of terminal disease.* Edward Arnold, London.

Stedeford, A. (1984) *Facing death: patients, families and professionals.* Heinemann, Oxford.

World Health Organization (1990) *Expert committee report*, series 804. WHO, Geneva.

Wilkinson, J. (1990) Ethics of euthanasia. *Palliative Care.* 4 81–6.

Appendix 1: Useful Addresses (as at 1994)

ACET (AIDS Care Education and Training)
PO Box 3693
London SW15 2BQ

Tel: 081 780 0400

Age Concern England
Astral House
1268 London Road
Norbury
London SW16 4EJ

Tel: 081 679 8000

Age Concern Wales
Fourth Floor
1 Cathedral Road
Cardiff CF1 9S

Tel: 0222 371 566

Alzheimer's Disease Society
Gordon House
10 Greencoat Place
London SW1P 1PH

Tel: 071 306 0606

Association of Hospice Administrators
Secretary: David Johnson
St Mary's Hospice
176 Raddlebarn Road
Selly Park
Birmingham B29 7DA

Tel: 021 472 1191

Association of Hospice Chaplains
Secretary: The Rev. Stuart Coates
Strathcarron Hospice
Randolph Hill
Denny
Stirling FK6 5HJ

Tel: 0324 826222

Association of Hospice Social Workers
Secretary: Howard Heyburn
Prospect Foundation
5 Church Place
Swindon SN1 5EH

Tel: 0793 616134

Association of Hospice Voluntary Service Co-ordinators
Secretary: Pam Warn
St Leonard's Hospice
185 Tadcaster Road
York YO2 2QL

Tel: 0904 708553

Association of Palliative Medicine
11 Westwood Road
Southampton SO2 1DL

Tel: 0703 672888

BACUP
3 Bath Place
Rivington Street
London EC2A 3JR

Tel: 071 613 2121

Breast Care and Mastectomy Association
15–19 Britten Street
London SW3 3TZ

Tel: 071 867 8275

British Colostomy Association (formerly Colostomy Welfare Group)
15 Station Road
Reading RG1 1LG

Tel: 0734 391537

British Diabetic Association
10 Queen Anne Street
London W1M 0BD

Tel: 071 323 1531

British Epilepsy Association
Anstey House
40 Hanover Square
Leeds LS3 1BE

Tel: 0532 439393

Cancerlink
17 Britannia Street
London WC1X 9JN

Tel: 071 833 2818

Cancer Relief Macmillan Fund
Anchor House
15–19 Britten Street
London SW3 3TZ

Tel: 071 351 7811

Child Poverty Action Group
1–5 Bath Street
London EC1V 9PY

Tel: 071 253 3406

The Compassionate Friends
53 North Street
Bristol BS3 1EN

Tel: 0272 539639

CRUSE
126 Sheen Road
Richmond
Surrey TW9 1UR

Tel: 081 940 4818

Disabled Living Foundation
380 Harrow Road
London W9 2HU

Tel: 071 289 6111

Help The Aged
St James' Walk
London EC1R 0BE

Tel: 071 253 1253

Help the Hospices
34–44 Britannia Street
London WC1X 9JG

Tel: 071 278 5668

Hospice Information Service
St Christopher's Hospice
51 Lawrie Park Road
Sydenham
London SE26 6DZ

Tel: 081 778 9525

International School for Cancer Care (ISCC)
Sir Michael Sobell House
Churchill Hospital
Oxford OX3 7LJ

Tel: 0865 225886

Leukaemia Research
c/o 20 Widdicombe Avenue
Canford Cliffs
Poole
Dorset BH14 9QW

Marie Curie Cancer Care
28 Belgrave Square
London SW1X 8QG

Tel: 071 736 6267

Multiple Sclerosis Society
25 Effie Road
Fulham
London SW6 1EE

Tel: 071 736 6267

National Association of Laryngectomy Clubs and Associates
Ground Floor
6 Rickett Street
Fulham
London SW6 1RU

Tel: 071 381 9993

The National Association of Widows
54–57 Allison Street
Digbeth
Birmingham B5 5TH

Tel: 021 643 8348

National Council for Hospice and Specialist Palliative Care Services
59 Bryanston Street
London W1A 2AZ

Tel: 071 611 1216/1153/1225

National Listening Library (Talking books and tapes)
12 Lant Street
London SE1 1QH

Tel: 071 407 9417

Nurse Managers' Forum
Royal College of Nursing
20 Cavendish Square
London W1M 0AB

Tel: 071 409 3333

One Parent Families
255 Kentish Town Road
London NW5 2LX

Tel: 071 267 1361

Palliative Care Centre (Trent)
Little Common Lane
Abbey Lane
Sheffield S11 9NE

Tel: 0742 620174

The Royal National Institute for the Blind
224–228 Great Portland Street
London W1N 6AA

Tel: 071 388 1266

The Royal National Institute for the Deaf
105 Gower Street
London WC1E 6AH

Tel: 071 387 8033

Sue Ryder Foundation Headquarters
Cavendish
Sudbury
Suffolk CO10 8AY

Tel: 0787 280252

St Christopher's Hospice
51 Lawrie Park Road
Sydenham
London NW5 2LX

Tel: 081 778 9252

St Joseph's Hospice
Mare Street
Hackney
London E8 4SA

Tel: 081 985 0861

The Samaritans
See local telephone book under 'S'

DHSS Leaflet D49 – "What to do after a death"
Enquiries should be addressed to DHSS Leaflet Unit, PO Box 21, Stanmore, HA7 1AY, or alternatively ring 071 972 2000 and ask for Leaflets Unit, Stanmore.

Appendix 2: Courses

Diploma in Palliative Medicine
One year, extramural, designed for doctors. Now available from:
University of Wales College of Medicine
Holme Tower
Marie Curie Centre
Bridgeman Road
Penarth
S Glamorgan CF6 2AW

Diploma/MSc in Psychosocial Palliative Medicine
University of Southampton
Dept of Social Work Studies
Southampton SO9 5NH
Diploma course also under preparation at Sheffield University (Palliative Care Centre, Trent) *see* Addresses.
   Many other courses, attachments, study days are available for professionals in the various disciplines of palliative care.
   For details contact:
- Help the Hospices
- Marie Curie Cancer Care

   For the relevant association see addresses.
   The larger hospices also provide a wide variety of courses.

English National Board of Nursing
Many courses available depending on needs and status.
ENB Careers
PO Box 356
Sheffield S8 0SJ

Macmillan Palliation in Advanced Cancer
(Mac Pac) a distance learning pack from Cancer Relief Macmillan Fund (*see* Addresses)

Marie Curie – Interaction Video Disc Teaching Packs
Marie Curie Memorial Foundation
Education Dept
Edenhall
11 Lyndhurst Gardens
Hampstead
London NW3 5NS

The Open University
Death & Dying (K260)
Milton Keynes MK7 6AA

Terminal Care Information Folder
Published by:
Royal College of General Practitioners
14 Princes Gate
London SW7 1PU

Journals

- Palliative Medicine – Edward Arnold
- Journal of Palliative Care – Centre for Bioethics, Montreal, Canada
- Journal of Pain and Symptom Management – Elsevier
- European Journal of Cancer Care – Blackwell Scientific Publications
- Progress in Palliative Care – Leeds Medical Information (University of Leeds)

Appendix 3: Possible indications for corticosteroids in terminal illness

Adjuvant Analgesic

1 Raised intracranial pressure
2 Nerve compression and neuropathic pain
3 Head and neck tumour, intrapelvic tumour, abdominal or retroperitoneal tumour
4 Hepatomegaly
5 Bone tumours
6 Lymphoedema

Respiratory Symptoms

1 Airways obstruction
2 Superior vena caval obstruction
3 Cough
4 Haemoptysis

Gastrointestinal Symptoms

1 Intestinal obstruction
2 Nausea and vomiting
3 Discharge from rectal tumour (via enema)
4 Anorexia and cachexia

Neurological Symptoms

1 Spinal cord compression (consider if incipient paraplegia)
2 Raised intracranial pressure
3 Carcinomatous neuromyopathy

Other

1 Enhance sense of well-being
2 Improve strength
3 Leucoerythroblastic anaemia
4 Reduce ureter/urethral obstruction due to tumour
5 Minimize toxic effect of radiation or chemotherapy
6 Allergic reaction
7 Reduce fever

Appendix 4: Approximate Oral Opioid Equivalents (24 hour doses)

Opioid	Conversion factor to oral morphine
Pentazocine	0.06
Codeine	0.08
Dihydrocodeine	0.1
Pethidine	0.125
Dextropropoxyphene	0.16
Dipipanone (in Diconal)	0.5
Morphine (oral)	1
Controlled release morphine	1
Diamorphine (oral)	1
Methadone	1
Dextromoramide	2
Phenazocine	5
Levorphanol	5
Hydromorphone (oral)	7.5
Buprenorphine	50
Hydromorphone (parenteral)	15
Morphine (parenteral)	2
Diamorphine (parenteral)	3
Fentanyl (transdermal) (for 72-hour dose)	Factor uncertain, under testing.

Appendix 5: Syringe Driver (eg Graseby MS16A)

Requirements

1 Prescription from doctor
2 Syringe driver
3 PP3 type battery
4 Appropriate syringe eg 10 ml Monoject
5 Graseby 100 cm infusion set (25 g needle)
6 Transparent dressing
7 OpSite or Blenderm tape
8 Antiseptic swab

Setting up the Syringe Driver

1 Full explanation of its purpose to patient and carers
2 Draw up medication and diluent
3 Connect infusion set to syringe. If this is a new infusion, prime tubing and needle with solution (less than 1.0 ml)
4 Insert battery and keep spare battery
5 Press start/test button. Machine available will produce a soft whirring and indicator light will flash on/off
6 Check correct rate is set. Graseby syringe drivers work in millimetres not millilitres. (Usually set is to deliver contents of syringe over 24 hours). Most 10 ml syringes give a fluid length of 48 mm, therefore 2 mm/hour.
7 Fit syringe with infusion tubing and needle to syringe driver. Place flange of syringe in slot provided and secure with rubber strap. Extra tape may be used to secure syringe
8 Fit plunger. Press white release button, then slide plunger assembly until it presses against syringe plunger inserting the cannula
9 If Graseby MS26 is being used, remember this syringe driver works in mm/day (24 hours). Therefore, set the fluid length of the syringe if a 24 hour infusion is required.

Inserting the Cannula

1 Choose a site for the butterfly needle. The most useful sites are the upper chest, outer aspect of upper arm, abdomen and thighs (never in an oedematous area)
2 Insert the needle at 45 degrees subcutaneously
3 Cover butterfly with transparent dressing. Anchor small circle of tubing to prevent 'pulling' on butterfly
4 Place clear plastic case into the holster and insert the pump into the case

Notes
Site should be checked daily and changed if area is inflamed, painful or lumpy
Start/test button may be used to deliver small extra dose, eg prior to changing a painful dressing
Light stops flashing when battery is low; pump will continue to operate for 24 hours after this
Battery lasts approximately six weeks
Battery lasts approximately 100 syringes

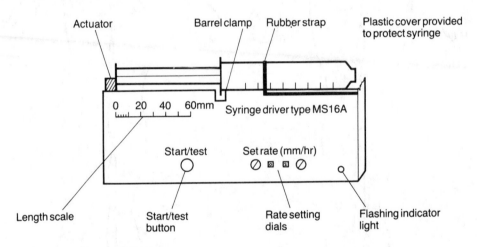

Figure 5.1: Graseby MS16A pump

Appendix 6

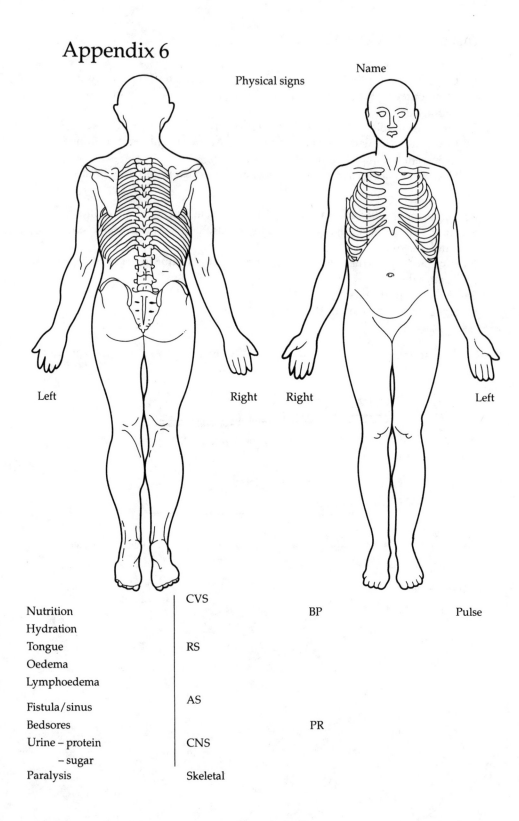

Physical signs

Name

Left

Right

Right

Left

Nutrition	CVS		BP		Pulse
Hydration					
Tongue	RS				
Oedema					
Lymphoedema					
Fistula/sinus	AS				
Bedsores			PR		
Urine – protein	CNS				
– sugar					
Paralysis	Skeletal				

Pain chart

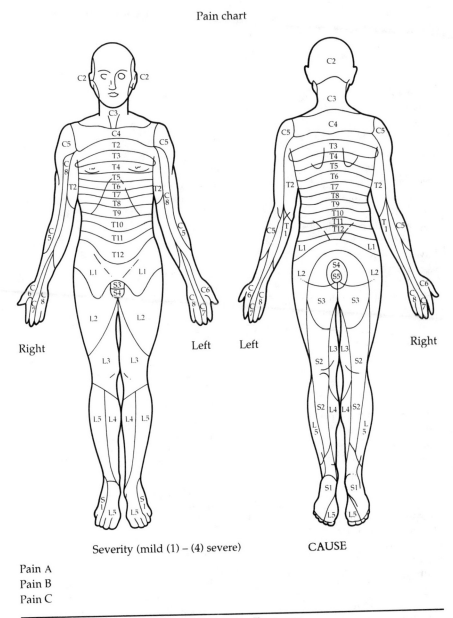

Severity (mild (1) – (4) severe)   CAUSE

Pain A
Pain B
Pain C

Problems   Treatment

Index